SpringerBriefs in Public Health

SpringerBriefs in Public Health present concise summaries of cutting-edge research and practical applications from across the entire field of public health, with contributions from medicine, bioethics, health economics, public policy, biostatistics, and sociology.

The focus of the series is to highlight current topics in public health of interest to a global audience, including health care policy; social determinants of health; health issues in developing countries; new research methods; chronic and infectious disease epidemics; and innovative health interventions.

Featuring compact volumes of 55 to 125 pages, the series covers a range of content from professional to academic. Possible volumes in the series may consist of timely reports of state-of-the art analytical techniques, reports from the field, snapshots of hot and/or emerging topics, literature reviews, and in-depth case studies. Both solicited and unsolicited manuscripts are considered for publication in this series.

Briefs are published as part of Springer's eBook collection, with millions of users worldwide. In addition, Briefs are available for individual print and electronic purchase.

Briefs are characterized by fast, global electronic dissemination, standard publishing contracts, easy-to-use manuscript preparation and formatting guidelines, and expedited production schedules. We aim for publication 8–12 weeks after acceptance.

Raman Bedi · Beatrice Merli · Esther Okorodudu · Nicole Gesare · Thuto Serufe Makara

Faith Communities and Global Health

Partnerships and Practice in the Global South

WFPHA World Federation of Public Health Associations

Springer

Raman Bedi
World Federation of Public Health
Associations (WFPHA)
Geneva, Switzerland

King's College London
London, UK

Esther Okorodudu
World Federation of Public Health
Associations (WFPHA)
Geneva, Switzerland

Thuto Serufe Makara
World Federation of Public Health
Associations (WFPHA)
Geneva, Switzerland

Beatrice Merli
World Federation of Public Health
Associations (WFPHA)
Geneva, Switzerland

Nicole Gesare
World Federation of Public Health
Associations (WFPHA)
Geneva, Switzerland

ISSN 2192-3698 ISSN 2192-3701 (electronic)
SpringerBriefs in Public Health
ISBN 978-3-032-29416-6 ISBN 978-3-032-29417-3 (eBook)
https://doi.org/10.1007/978-3-032-29417-3

This Springer imprint is published by the registered company Springer Nature Switzerland AG
The registered company address is: Gewerbestrasse 11, 6330 Cham, Switzerland

This book is dedicated to my parents,
Mr. Satya-Pal Bedi and Mrs. Raj Bedi,
who left India to seek a better life for
themselves and their children.
Although leaving India, the country never
quite left them.
Raman Bedi

A zia Bebe per aver chiamato,
e a Lorenzo per aver risposto,
in un giorno di primavera.
Beatrice Merli

To my parents,
whose guidance, sacrifices and
encouragement
have shaped by journey of faith.
Esther Okorodudu

To my parents,
my greatest supporters,
who always reminded me that
words have the power to change the world.
Nicole Gesare

To my parents,
who first showed me the healing power of
faith.
Thuto Serufe Makara

Foreword

Since the earliest times, humans have sought to explain the world that surrounds them through a variety of explanatory frameworks. Even today, many fundamental questions remain unresolved, prompting individuals to turn to diverse systems of belief. Among these enduring concerns, health has always occupied a central place in human reflection, shaping experiences from birth to death and everything in between.

In this book, the authors explore the links between belief systems—particularly faith-based ones—and health, with a special focus on public health. This relationship, marked by a long and intricate history, is presented through a balanced analysis of mutual influence.

Its roots are traced to prehistoric healing practices and the rise of monotheistic religions, where moral imperatives gradually contributed to the development of early public health concepts. The contemporary parallels between religious ethics and public health mandates are explored further, offering a nuanced perspective on critiques that portray public health as a "nanny state," sometimes perceived as a form of moral prescription resembling religious doctrine.

The book also considers how religious traditions and public health have shaped one another over time. In particular, it examines how classical monotheistic religions have reinforced patriarchal hierarchies through scriptural interpretation and institutional authority. These dynamics remain highly relevant today, as they continue to be invoked in the justification of gender-based violence and feminicide. A comparable analysis is extended to the field of mental health.

Attention is also given to the charitable activities of religious organizations in low- and middle-income countries, many of which have historical ties to colonial contexts. Their contributions to fragile or under-resourced health systems are highlighted. This discussion could be strengthened by further examination of the structural factors underlying disparities between these countries and high-income settings, as well as the specific role faith-based organizations play within these broader inequalities.

Overall, the volume provides a solid foundation for deeper inquiry into the complex relationship between faith-based systems and public health. It serves as an excellent introduction to a vast and multifaceted field. Future research might address the expanding "market" of contemporary healers—both digital and in-person—as well as the commercialization of traditional practices such as yoga within the global health economy. Additional questions arise regarding the interaction between so-called alternative medicine, with its underlying belief frameworks, and conventional biomedicine. The intersections of health and faith are rich and varied, offering ample material for a compelling follow-up volume.

February 2026

Bettina Borisch
World Federation of Public Health Associations (WFPHA)
Geneva, Switzerland

Preface

This book emerges from a deeply personal conviction that has shaped my professional life: that faith communities represent one of the world's most underutilized assets in advancing global health equity.

My own journey began unexpectedly, during my university years at Bristol, where a Christian conversion profoundly reoriented my understanding of purpose, service, and the inherent dignity of every person. What started as a personal, spiritual awakening evolved into a professional calling—to bridge worlds that too often operate in parallel: the world of evidence-based public health and the world of faith-based community action.

As I assumed leadership roles, I have repeatedly witnessed the same paradox. Faith communities constitute the oldest and most extensive health infrastructure in human history, yet they remain marginalized in mainstream public health discourse. In many settings across the Global South, faith-based organizations provide a large proportion of health services, particularly in rural and underserved areas. They enjoy levels of community trust that government systems often struggle to achieve. They mobilize volunteers, resources, and social capital at scales that would be the envy of any public health program.

Yet how often do our academic curricula seriously engage with faith as a social determinant of health? How often do our public health strategies genuinely partner with—rather than merely utilize—faith communities? How often do we acknowledge that for millions of people worldwide, faith is not peripheral but central to their understanding of health, healing, and human flourishing?

This book does not advocate for a particular religious tradition, nor does it uncritically romanticize faith communities. Rather, it seeks to examine rigorously and honestly what happens when public health systems and faith communities move beyond transactional relationships toward genuine partnership. It explores historical foundations, contemporary challenges, and sustainable models for integration. Most importantly, it centers voices and experiences from the Global South, where the intersection of faith and health is not theoretical but lived reality.

The timing is critical. As we navigate the post-pandemic era, the limitations of purely technocratic approaches to health have become painfully apparent. The

COVID-19 pandemic revealed both the fragility of our health systems and the resilience of community-based responses, many of them faith-driven. As we work toward Universal Health Coverage and the health-related Sustainable Development Goals, we cannot afford to overlook the potential of faith communities as partners in this endeavor.

My role as incoming President of the World Federation of Public Health Associations (WFPHA) has reinforced this conviction. In traveling extensively across Asia, Africa, and Latin America, I have encountered countless examples of innovative faith-health partnerships addressing topics from maternal mortality, through non-communicable diseases, to mental health. These are not marginal experiments; they represent scalable, sustainable models that deserve serious scholarly attention and policy consideration.

This book brings together diverse voices to examine these partnerships from multiple perspectives. Some chapters are celebratory; others are appropriately critical. This diversity is intentional. The integration of faith and health in the Global South is complex, contested, and contextual. Any honest examination must reflect that complexity.

I am deeply grateful to all the contributing authors, who have brought intellectual rigor, practical wisdom, and personal courage to this project. I thank Springer for their willingness to publish a work that challenges conventional boundaries. I acknowledge the countless faith-based health workers—many unnamed and unrecognized—whose daily service inspired this book. And I thank my colleagues at the Christian Dental Fellowship, King's College London, and WFPHA, who have supported and shaped my thinking over many years.

This book is offered in the hope that it will inspire more equitable, more effective, and more humane approaches to global health approaches that recognize faith communities not as obstacles to overcome or tools to deploy, but as partners in the shared work of healing.

London, UK
February 2026

Raman Bedi

Acknowledgments We are grateful to the staff of the World Federation of Public Health Associations and the member National Public Health Associations for their help and support.

Competing Interests The authors have no competing interests to declare that are relevant to the content of this manuscript.

About This Book

This book emerges from a conviction shaped by experience, history, and repeated observation: faith communities are among the oldest institutional foundations of the global health system and remain structurally embedded in many health systems across the Global South.

This conviction has been reinforced through engagement with the World Federation of Public Health Associations (WFPHA), which brings together national public health associations from more than 130 countries. In conversations across Africa, Asia, Latin America, and Europe, one lesson has recurred with consistency: technical capacity alone does not guarantee public health effectiveness. Health systems function within social ecosystems, and those ecosystems are often structured by institutions of faith.

Modern public health often narrates its own development as a progression from religious charity to secular governance; yet historical evidence tells a more complex story. Hospitals and community-based care systems were built within religious frameworks long before the rise of modern state health systems. Secularization did not erase these infrastructures, rather, it reclassified them as peripherical.

In the twenty-first century, global health is increasingly driven by technological innovation. Yet technology alone does not produce health outcomes, which depend on what tools are available as much as on how communities engage with them.

Across epidemics, from HIV/AIDS, through Ebola to COVID-19, technical innovations were developed and deployed. Community engagement was pursued by leveraging on faith actors, who were not integrated systematically into preparedness planning and early management. This reflects deeper assumptions about what counts as legitimate health infrastructure.

In many regions, faith-inspired institutions operate healthcare networks that are intertwined with national health systems. At the same time, measurement gaps, fragmented reporting, and governance frameworks often obscure their full contribution and undermine appropriate financing, planning, and integration. This further supports the secular conceptualization of authority and legitimacy in broader health systems.

The central argument of this book is therefore pragmatic rather than theological. Technological innovation is necessary for development, but engagement determines its effectiveness. In contexts where religion shapes social norms and interpretations of illness, leveraging religious institutions is a strategic choice for strengthening compliance and accelerating progress toward shared development goals.

The chapters that follow examine this argument across history, emergency response, regional service provision, mental health, gender, and sustainable development. Taken together, they suggest that the future of global health will not be determined solely by technical innovation, but by how systems navigate plural sources of meaning.

Contents

About the Authors

Raman Bedi is Emeritus Professor at King's College London, United Kingdom, and President-elect of the World Federation of Public Health Associations (WFPHA). As former Chief Dental Officer for England, his career has spanned academic leadership, public health policy, and international health development. His research focuses on transcultural oral health, non-communicable disease (NCD) management, and health equity. He is President of the Christian Dental Fellowship (CDF).

Following his life changing conversion, he served ten years on the General Synod of the Church of England and was founding chair of its Race and Community Affairs Committee. His strong Christian faith informs his public health approach today.

Beatrice Merli is an MSc student at Bocconi University, Italy. Her research focuses on Public-Private Partnerships (PPPs) and social infrastructure investments, with a specialization in global health financing from the Graduate Institute of International and Development Studies. She is a research intern at the World Federation of Public Health Associations (WFPHA) and volunteers with Working for Wasa. Raised Catholic, she identifies as a spiritual person.

Esther Okorodudu is an MSc student in Public Health, with interests in epidemiology, health equity, and the intersection of faith, gender, and well-being. As a research intern at the World Federation of Public Health Associations (WFPHA), she explores how religious communities influence health practice and policy. Raised in a Christian household, guided by her mother's faith, her faith shapes her approach to public health.

Nicole Gesare is an MSc student in Public Health at Umeå University, Sweden. Her research interests are in health equity and in migration, culture and religion as determinants of health and well-being. She is a research intern at the World Federation of Public Health Associations (WFPHA) and at Unisanté, Switzerland. Raised Anglican, she identifies as spiritual but not a practicing Christian.

Thuto Serufe Makara completed an MSc at the London School of Hygiene and Tropical Medicine, United Kingdom, and will begin her PhD studies shortly. As an intern at the World Federation of Public Health Associations (WFPHA), she has published several academic papers. Her research spans cancer and the role of faith in promoting well-being. A practicing Christian, her faith drives her commitment to communicating the healing power of faith.

Abbreviations

ADRA	Adventist Relief Agency
ADS	AIDS Data System
AKDN	Aga Khan Development Network
ARENELA+	African Network of Religious Leaders Living with or Personally Affected by HIV and AIDS
ARDF	Anglican Relief and Development Funds
BGR	Buddhist Global Relief
CBT	Cognitive Behavioural Therapy
CDC	Centers for Disease Control and Prevention
CEDAW	Convention on the Elimination of All Forms of Discrimination Against Women
CFBI	Center for Faith and Opportunity Initiatives at USAID
CHAI	Christian Health Association of India
CHAM	Christian Health Association of Malawi
CHAMC	Christian Health Asset Mapping Consortium
CHAN	Christian Health Association of Nigeria
CHAZ	Christian Health Association of Zambia
CIFA	Christian Interfaith Foundation for Public Health in Africa
CMMB	Catholic Medical Mission Board
CRC	Convention on the Rights of the Child
CSSC	Christian Social Services Commission
DALYs	Disability-Adjusted Life Years
DSD	Disorders of Sex Development
ECTs	Ebola Treatment Centres
EMRO	Eastern Mediterranean Region
FBOs	Faith-Based Organizations
FGM	Female Genital Mutilation
FIIs	Faith-Inspired Institutions
GOARN	Global Outbreak Alert and Response Network
HIPC	Heavily Indebted Poor Countries
IBRO	International Buddhist Relief Organization

IIRO	International Islamic Relief Organization
JLI	Joint Learning Initiative on Faith and Local Communities
KEWASNET	Kenya Water and Sanitation Civil Society Network
LGB	Lesbian, Gay, Bisexual
MDGs	Millennium Development Goals
MHGAP	Mental Health Gap Action Programme
MIND	Mindfulness Intervention to Study the Neurobiology of Depression
MSF	Médecins Sans Frontières
NCDs	Non-Communicable Diseases
NIFAA	Nigerian Interfaith Action Association
OOPs	Out-of-Pocket Payments
PARD	International Partnership on Religion and Sustainable Development
PPPs	Public-Private Partnerships
PTSD	Post-Traumatic Stress Disorder
RCBT	Religiously integrated Cognitive Behavioural Therapy
SACBC	Southern African Catholic Bishops' Conference
SACC	South African Council of Churches
SCPs	State–Church Partnerships
SDGs	Sustainable Development Goals
SLAs	Service Level Agreements
SSA	Sub-Saharan Africa
TIP	Tanzania Interfaith Partnership
TM	Traditional Medicine
UCMB	Uganda Catholic Medical Bureau
UHC	Universal Health Coverage
UN IATF-R	UN Interagency Task Force on Religion and Sustainable Development
UPMB	Uganda Protestant Medical Bureau
WASH	Water, Sanitation and Hygiene
WCC	World Council of Churches
WFDD	World Faiths Development Dialogue
WHO	World Health Organization
YLD	Years Lived with Disability
YLL	Years of Life Lost

Religious Foundations of Public Health

1 Introduction

Since before modern public health systems existed, disease prevention, as well as care for the sick and dying, was largely provided by religious institutions, which contributed to the establishment of formal public health infrastructure. This connection between faith and health has been constant across human civilizations, either via ancient priest-physicians, temple healers, or monastic caregivers.

This continuity challenges the widespread assumption that public health emerged primarily through secular modernity. Long before epidemiology and state-based administration formalized health governance, religious institutions had already institutionalized care, regulated communal behavior, and structured collective responsibility for well-being. Modern public health systems therefore did not arise in isolation from religion, but evolved from frameworks in which moral authority and organizational capacity were already embedded.

This chapter narrates the deep-rooted relationship between religion and health, with the purpose of pointing out how public health stems from ancient religious practices and how religious institutions supported the emergence of public health systems and infrastructure across the globe.

2 Indigenous Models of Health Care

Long before the establishment of formal public health systems, healing practices and spiritual beliefs were intertwined.

R. Bedi et al., *Faith Communities and Global Health*,
SpringerBriefs in Public Health, https://doi.org/10.1007/978-3-032-29417-3_1

Visual evidence from cave complexes in Southern Africa during the Paleolithic period (c. 30,000–10,000 BCE) denounces the presence of Shamanism in early societies. Indeed, according to Price (2001), most of the African rock art is a representation of Shaman's—the religious leaders of communities, who acted as mediators between the sky, earth, and underground and were thought to have the ability to connect them—visions, which were accomplished via a tranche dance, special curing rituals, viewing rock art and dreams (Price, 2001). Kolankaya-Bostanci (2014) complements this interpretation by stating that paintings represented Shamanistic rituals as well.

To our analysis, it is interesting to notice that the second method in which shamans achieved insights into spiritual things was used when a person was deemed to be very sick; in these circumstances, shamans looked into the body of a patient, identified the cause of the illness, removed it by the laying of hands, attracted it to their own bodies, and then expelled it via a hole in the back of the neck—visible to shamans only. Some shamans became renowned for their curing ability and were summoned from afar communities to perform their exams; this way, they sustained communication between distant camps. Overall, shamans used their visions for various purposes, among which causing rain to fall and guiding the movements of antelope so that they run into the hunters' ambush (Price, 2001).

With the Neolithic transition to sedentism (c. 10,000–3000 BCE), ritual life became spatially anchored; participation to it was enlarged and increasingly organized. Shamans' costumes were invested with several layers of meaning and amplified their performance; for example, the fringes of their coats allowed the shaman to penetrate into the upper and lower spheres of the universe. Overall, the shaman's body itself became a stage on which cosmology was displayed.

By the early modern period, Siberian shamans were ethnographically documented. Under colonial expansion, they hybridized with local traditions, like the *Sangomas* in Southern Africa and the *Curanderos* in Latin America. These historical evolutions show that, long before secular institutions formalized public health systems, ritual authority structured responses to individual and social disruption, with the purpose of preserving moral and social order. Across regions and cultures, spiritual practices emphasized the *interconnection* of body, spirit, and community.

These practices were not merely symbolic or explanatory frameworks for illness; they constituted organized mechanisms for regulating social cohesion and collective well-being. Ritual specialists mediated conflict, reinforced communal norms, and managed perceived threats to physical and moral order. In this sense, indigenous healing systems functioned as early forms of health governance embedded within cosmology rather than state administration.

Sangomas in Southern Africa. Sangomas are mediums and ritual specialists. Individuals can self-declare to be Sangomas, for example on a hereditary basis, or be chosen by ancestors to become Sangomas. The process of being called and then initiated is called *thwasa,* and is characterized by symptoms such as psychosis, severe headaches, abdominal pain, shoulder, and neck complaints which vanish once the student accepts the initiation process. The latter is about creating a relationship between the student and ancestors, and is essential to acquiring healing power and performing tasks (Cumes, 2013).

Health consultations by Sangomas occur in a healing hut (*ndumba*) with a formal protocol, which involves removing shoes, kneeling, clapping to greet the spirits, burning *mphepho*—a plant with a pleasant smell—and lighting candles. Diagnosis is performed through trances—where the healer communicates with ancestors—and divination with bones—where bones are cast and read (Cumes, 2013).

Treatment consists of *muti*, a mixture of plants, animal, mineral substances administered in baths, steams, or incisions; these have little pharmacological action, as their main effectiveness derives by the fact that they are administered by the Sangoma. For malevolent influences, Sangomas may perform *femba* (exorcism) on people and houses to remove pollution and restore communal order (Cumes, 2013).

Curanderismo. From the Spanish verb *curar* (to heal), curanderismo is a healing tradition found in Mexican American communities. Its intellectual base rests on the distinction between illnesses of a natural origin and of supranatural cause. In this framework, a person may suffer from diabetes as a biomedical metabolic disorder, treatable by physicians, and from a form triggered by spiritual imbalance or malevolent intervention, which require treatment by Curanderos. Curanderos operate through what is described as *el don*—a gift of healing—historically understood as divinely granted but increasingly interpreted as an innate human capacity developed through training.

The theoretical structure of curanderismo is organized into three levels: the material (*nivel material*), the spiritual (*nivel espiritual*), and the mental (*nivel mental*); each level involves distinct forms of diagnosis, intervention, and authority (Trotter, 1996).

Most Curanderos have the gift for working at the material level, whose related interventions can be subdivided into physical and supernatural manipulations. In the former, the Curandero manipulates substances—herbs, foods, oils, candles, eggs, animals, and religious objects—to restore balance (e.g., tea to reduce fever). In the latter, rituals support cleansing; for example, a patient might be swept with lemon, basil, or garlic that absorb negative vibrations, while prayers are recited (Trotter, 1996). The spiritual level is parallel to shaman healing, as it requires individuals to enter an altered state of consciousness and make contact with the spirit world by opening one's mind to spirit voices, or sending one's spirit out of the body to gain knowledge at a distance. The mental level is the least commonly encountered; here the Curandero sends mental vibrations directed toward the patient to influence his physical and behavioral states—for example, to retard the progression of diseases, or to limit alcoholism (Trotter, 1996). Across all three levels, illness reflects imbalance across interconnected domains (Maduro, 1983).

By framing illness as imbalance across material, spiritual, and social dimensions, these systems embedded health within a broader moral and communal structure. Authority over healing was inseparable from authority over social meaning, demonstrating that the management of illness operated simultaneously as management of collective order. Such configurations reveal that structured health responses long preceded the formalization of public health within modern states.

3 The Proto-Public Health Function of Religion

In prehistoric societies, healing knowledge was transmitted orally by ritual specialists. With the rise of urban societies in Mesopotamia in the third millennium BCE, healing knowledge began to be written down in cuneiform tablets (Markham, 2010). Such documents provide evidence of the combination of incantations and medical recipes used by the Babylonians to treat the different psychological and physical symptoms of patients. Consequently, practitioners started to follow recorded instructions that integrated personal experience. Eventually writings on healing theory supported the institutionalization of such practices within early urban civilizations.

Although the extent to which Egyptian medicine functioned as a fully centralized state system remains debated, available evidence suggests that medical practice was closely embedded within temple and court institutions. An entourage of doctors specialized in public health surrounded the *Pharaoh* and promoted hygiene and prevention practices among the population (Rosso, 2023). From the first Dynasty onward, such professional figures were trained by priests via theoretical and practical classes, offered in temples. Priests also managed the process of updating existing medical scriptures, which was also performed in sacred places (Rosso, 2023). As treatment, administrative authorities promoted bathing, shaving, regulated diet, and water control, shaping sanitation practices and behavioral codes that contributed to population well-being, even if not conceptualized as "public health" in modern epidemiological terms.

Compared to Egyptians, who reinforced the unity of doctrine, Ancient Greek medicine was a compilation of divergent theories and practices in constant expansion (Rosso, 2023). This is clear when looking at the evolution of the activities performed in Asclepieia, the healing sanctuaries dedicated to Asclepios—the physician-demigod who treated wounded soldiers during Homer's Trojan War. Indeed, with the passage of time and increasing emphasis on real-world medicine, Asclepieia began employing physicians who could supplement their priests' mystical curatives. Patients would make pilgrimages to such temples and pursue a holistic, healthcare treatment based on spiritual and medical care. Preliminary procedures—including exercise, massages and fasting—were followed by specific medical or surgical treatments, after which patients spent the night in one of the sanctuary's sacred buildings, where they would wait for the God to enter their dreams and heal them (Pavli & Maltezou, 2024).

Taken together, these early civilizations demonstrate that religion *organized responses* to illness, combining moral authority with administrative capacity. The subsequent emergence of hospitals under Christian and Islamic governance should therefore be understood not as a rupture from religious care, but as its institutional consolidation.

4 Expansion of Hospitals and Progressive Secularization across Europe

From the fourth century onward, Christian communities began to *formalize* charitable assistance into permanent institutions; this formalization marks a shift from dispersed acts of charity to organized healthcare models, later attributed to secular public health systems. Box 1 explores the role of the monastic movement over this process.

The St. Basil's hospital of *Caesarea*, founded between 368 and 370 CE, first embodied the Christian model of hospitalization according to Riva and Cesana (2013), who describe it as similar to a city, with streets separating pavilion, convalescent homes, and residences for attendants, nurses, and physicians. While agreeing on some of the physical features of the facility, Caner (2018) notes that the institution functioned as a leprosarium rather than a hospital, intended primarily for the long-term care of persons afflicted with severe leprosy. Both interpretations are meaningful, given that the second builds on an ideological priority of the founder to care for lepers as the most dramatic symbol of poverty under monastic impulses.

Eventually, some historians believe that Christian hospitality influenced the development of healing centers in countries under Islamic control. In contrast, Dols (1987) argues that early Islamic hospitals were shaped by Persian administrative models and their professionalization of medicine, which determined that *bimaritans* functioned as centers for secular clinical practice and medical instruction—rather than religiously influenced, welfare complexes. As a result, Islamic hospitals were private medical institutions run by highly placed government officials and funded via imperial patronage (Dols, 1987). Riva & Cesana, 2013) add that *bimaritans* also worked as centers of medical education for students from Europe and the far east, regardless of their religious beliefs.

Box 1 The monastic movement

The monastic movement emerged during the Early Middle Ages and, in the following centuries, developed into the largest institution in Europe taking care for the sick. In England alone, the number of monasteries rose to approximately one thousand; nearly every house maintained its own infirmary, and additional five hundred were managed and staffed by monks and nuns (Furniss, 1968). The density of this network enabled religious care to reach into urban and rural society.

Monastic life was structured around a comprehensive healing regimen covering prevention of illness, treatment of the sick, and preparation for death; most importantly, it fully integrated care of the body and soul, as care for the two was regarded as indivisible. In this sense, monasteries actively supported an integrated understanding of health.

Communal life in the reformed orders followed the rule of St Benedict, which disciplined the body through celibacy, fasting, and physical exercise—as well as prayer, study, talk, and sleep. Recreation in green spaces was also considered important; for example, walking in the monastic orchards, vineyards, and gardens helped rebalance the humors (Gilchrist, 2020).

The Benedictine emphasis on hospitality and charity extended this regimen beyond the cloister. Monasteries operated infirmaries at their gates and hospitals founded by ecclesiastics, aristocrats, and later merchants and guilds. Both institutions combined prayer and basic nursing care, differing primarily in emphasis rather than function. These were supported by impressive collections of medical texts—from the Ancient Greek to Islamic pharmacological texts.

In the end, medieval monasticism constituted a durable and replicable institutional system that structured healthcare and welfare across Europe. The scale, density, and continuity of these networks meant that monastic institutions effectively functioned as decentralized health systems.

In the Middle Ages, the Protestant Reformation led to the restructuring of religious institutions across Europe; in some cases, this determined the closure of monastic orders, along the hospitals they ran. Importantly, the emergence of civic and guild-based hospitals did not represent a rejection of religious health governance, but an adaptation of its institutional logic within expanding urban economies. Organizational forms originally embedded in ecclesiastical charity were reconfigured within civic administration, preserving structural continuity beneath apparent secular transition.

Adding to this, the interest in maintaining the health of citizens to preserve economic productivity and a well-functioning military nudged noblemen and kings to donate the wealth they had accumulated via commerce to support the expansion of city hospitals (Riva & Cesana, 2013). The guilds—associations of craftsmen and merchants in medieval cities—also collected funds for the relief of their sick members, building their own health facilities or paying other institutions for their accommodation and treatment. Such community-based initiatives complemented the religious-based ones and supported the emergence of hospitals under civic models.

From the thirteenth century on, the internal organization of such facilities evolved. Hospitals were structured around permanent medical staff and regulated procedures of admission and care, while religious members continued to provide spiritual assistance. As Henderson (2001) emphasizes, this dual aspect of hospitality was preserved in the Italian city-states of the Renaissance period, which continued to take care of the body and the soul under Christian influence. While rooted in religious charity, hospitals there functioned within a civic framework in which health care became a collective responsibility.

Later, the Enlightenment emphasis on the power of reason and science further sustained the transformation of hospitals into *medicalized spaces*. This intellectual shift narrowed the conceptual frame of health, privileging measurable outcomes and biomedical intervention over the integrated moral and communal dimensions that had previously structured care. While advances in clinical rationality strengthened treatment effectiveness, they also contributed to the gradual repositioning of religious institutions from systemic architects of health to supplementary actors within emerging state-based governance models. According to Balboni (2018), the fact hospitals' performance was assessed via mortality rates denounces the practical shift that invested healthcare facilities in the period, as their original role was to act as caregivers on the patient's journey into the next life. Yet, increasing wealth disparities indirectly resulted in a preservation of the original, religious hospital's role to care for the less advantaged. Indeed, Imhof (1977) confirms that hospitals welcomed lower-class members who (i) were either professionally secure or benefited from charity, and (ii) waited until the disease progressed to get cured; the better off could afford to be cured frequently at home.

5 The Educative Role of Religion in Africa and Latin America

Until the seventeenth century, missions in Africa were predominantly Portuguese and Catholic. The Portuguese were the first Europeans to establish small trading posts along the African coasts to conduct business with the native populations in exchange for natural resources. Their colonial initiatives were aided by the Church, as commerce and religion came together. To this point, Levi (2009) cites Johnston (1966) to recall that Portuguese priests and Jesuit fathers accompanied most of the early expeditions to Africa. Initially, those who converted did so more out of commercial need than because of a true desire for salvation (Levi, 2009), as converting meant entering into a sociopolitical alliance with the colonizers.

In the attempt to explain to local populations the European and Christian values, religious missions had to understand and use the local languages effectively to communicate with the people. Missionaries had to be trained on local languages and cultures before embarking on missions; to support this task, a press exclusively devoted to the printing of works dedicated to evangelization in these countries was founded. Once ready, a missionary could give his sermons in the local language(s) and guide the local populations in the conversion process (Levi, 2009).

The first systematic study of Albanian, Arabic, Armenian, Chaldean, Ethiopian, Georgian, Greek, Hebrew, Mbundu, Nahuatl, Syriac, and Wallach was commissioned for the sole purpose of helping the evangelization process (Dahlmann, 1891 in Levi, 2009). Eventually, this involved the writing of glossaries, alphabets, grammar, and arithmetical books, which started to be employed in the education field along with history and geography books, whose production followed. The translation of the Bible, Prayers, and Hymns into African languages took many years, and contributed to the development of an education closely intertwined with religion, so that it is impossible to overestimate the importance of the Bible in African society (Pawliková-Vilhanová, 2007).

In the following centuries, Protestant and Anglican initiatives joined up the Christian ones, whose revival after the French Revolution and Napoleonic Wars came in the late eighteenth century. In that period, Pawliková-Vilhanová (2007) states that the expansion of the missionary movement was influenced by a growing conception of Christian responsibility for the regeneration of African people after slavery.

In most regions of Sub-Saharan Africa outside the reach of Islam, where Christian missionaries had to promote their faith as a superior alternative, Africans were introduced to written literature through Christian propaganda (Pawliková-Vilhanová, 2007). The initiation of these populations to literature was conceptualized as flexible to local traditions, under the motto "transforming Africa by the Africans" (Lavigerie, 1874). However, the praxis of the missionary initiative often turned out to be different from its original conception (Pawliková-Vilhanová, 2007).

Early mission schools placed a heavy emphasis on religion. Most schools provided only basic education to ensure the proper inculcation of Christian principles, as well as Western values—which were promoted as superior and soon imposed the abandonment of local customs, such as polygamy. The conversion to Christian and Western values was facilitated by the distance between the school facilities and the homes of students (Pawliková-Vilhanová, 2007). By merging local traditions and Western influences, Africans themselves were instrumental in the formation of a new *cultural synthesis* (Pawliková-Vilhanová, 2007). Crucially, this synthesis did not dissolve religious institutions into secular governance; rather, it positioned them as enduring intermediaries between communities and formal administrative systems. In many contexts, religious networks became structurally intertwined with education and health delivery, shaping patterns of authority that persisted beyond the colonial period.

Today, there is extensive evidence on the long-term impact that the historical presence of European missionaries had on the economic development of the countries of destination. Nunn (2014) states that in Africa, both Protestant and Catholic missions increased the educational attainment of descendants via altered importance of education and proximity to educational infrastructure. The effect of education at the ethnicity level is reported to be three times the magnitude of the effect of physical proximity to the village, suggesting a mechanism where educational investments resonate across generations. Other studies in the African context report that protestant missions supported democracy (Lankina & Getachew, 2012).

In Latin America, Caicedo (2017) states that municipalities where the Jesuits converted the indigenous people exhibited 10%–15% higher literacy rates in 2017, as well as 10% higher per capita income. The author explains the effects on human capital and educational attainment via structural transformation and technology adoption; indeed, Jesuit missions supported a shift from agriculture—thanks to higher agricultural productivity—into manufacturing and services.

Overall, religious organizations were central actors in the diffusion of education in both Africa and Latin America. By introducing literacy and new forms of knowledge, they contributed to shaping the institutional and cultural foundations of the societies that later emerged, contributing to their configurations today. Their investments in education enabled technology adoption and structural transformation; eventually, they contributed to the empowerment and development of generations of Africans and Latinos. Such legacies complicate narratives that portray modernization as a purely secular process and highlight the institutional entanglement of faith and development. Beyond education, religious organizations were equally central to the provision of medical care, particularly in rural and underserved areas, as Box 2 explores.

Box 2 Missionary medicine in Sub-Saharan Africa (SSA)
Missionary organizations have historically played a central role in the provision of education and medical care.

Initially, mission hospitals missionary hospitals as primary health systems in rural and underserved areas long before national ministries of health developed comparable reach. They focused on curative medicine and posed large attention on maternal and child health. For example, in colonial Tanganyika, mission antenatal clinics outnumbered those constructed by the government after independence (Adu-Gyamfi et al., 2020). Missionaries also trained local nurses, midwives, and vaccinators; by around 1925, approximately 500 indigenous nurses had been trained across 116 hospitals and 366 dispensaries on the continent (Adu-Gyamfi et al., 2020). The target population of these facilities consisted in the most vulnerable, including the poor, women, children, and individuals with stigmatized diseases.

Over time, missionary hospitals diversified their funding sources from patient fees. In contemporary contexts, financing may include partnerships with NGOs, international donors, bilateral agencies, and state subventions. Some mission hospitals now operate under formal service agreements with governments, or receive public funding while maintaining denominational oversight. In Kenya, approximately 23% of hospital beds are provided by missionary hospitals; in Cameroon, faith-based institutions provide roughly 40% of national healthcare services (Adu-Gyamfi et al., 2020).

Staffing patterns have also changed. Early mission hospitals were often staffed by a single expatriate doctor, with assistants and religious actors; gradually, trained local personnel replaced them.

Today, governments increasingly rely on mission hospitals for program implementation, including vaccination campaigns, and infectious disease control. During the 2014 Ebola outbreak, faith-based health networks in Liberia and neighboring countries played a significant role in training healthcare workers, providing personal protective equipment, and maintaining service delivery where government facilities had closed. Mission hospitals also participated in HIV/AIDS awareness and treatment programs.

Overall, mission hospitals have transitioned from early missionary outposts to structurally embedded components of many sub-Saharan African health systems, supporting service delivery, personnel training, and public health initiatives over time.

6 Conclusion

Across historical contexts, faith groups acted as early system-builders, providing organizational capacity, social trust networks, and moral authority. This role was deeply embedded in Christian theology itself, which placed care for the sick and vulnerable at the heart of its mission. Early Christian communities distinguished themselves through organized acts of compassion, which translated institutionally into leprosaria and hospitals that later shaped both European and global health infrastructures.

In Africa and Latin America, religious institutions were central also to the diffusion of education and literacy. They created durable infrastructure and embedded new forms of knowledge within community life.

Over time, a process of progressive secularization unfolded. In the post-Enlightenment era, religion was increasingly separated from governance and science, and hospitals originally embedded in religious charity evolved into medicalized spaces integrated into public systems. Eventually, religion was repositioned at the margins of public health governance.

Recognizing that the architecture of modern public health systems was co-produced through religious initiative—later formalized under secular governance—allows to highlight faith-based institutions as foundational contributors to health-care development. Their influential role is still enormous today, as proven by the last waves of epidemics and pandemics (e.g., Ebola, HIV/AIDS, COVID-19), where their collaboration has been essential to enhance compliance beyond secular communication strategies.

Reframing the history of public health in this way has contemporary implications. When modern governance models treat faith-based institutions as supplementary or symbolic partners, they risk overlooking the institutional depth and social authority that these actors historically possessed and, in many regions, continue to hold. The narrative of rupture between religion and public health obscures the layered evolution of health systems and may contribute to the persistent under-integration of religious infrastructures in policy design.

Public health governance would benefit from more systematic and structured engagement with faith-based institutions. Integrating their social capital, community legitimacy, and organizational networks into formal public health planning can strengthen resilience, improve outreach, and enhance the effectiveness of future health interventions.

References

Adu-Gyamfi, S., Kuusaana, M. M., Darkwa, B. D., et al. (2020). The changing landscape of Mission medicine and hospitals in sub-Saharan Africa. *Christian Journal for Global Health, 7*(5), 65–81. https://doi.org/10.15566/cjgh.v7i5.417

Balboni, M. (2018). *The evolution of the hospital: History of medicine and religion, hospitals, palliative care. Religion and spirituality in health and medicine.* Harvard University. https://archive.blogs.harvard.edu/healthandreligion/2018/02/27/evolutionofthehospital/. Accessed on February 10, 2026

Caicedo, F. V. (2017). The Mission: Human capital transmission, economic persistence, and culture in South America. *Quarterly Journal of Economics, 134*(1), 507–556.

Caner, D. (2018). Not a hospital but a leprosarium: Basil's Basilias and an early byzantine concept of the deserving poor. *Dumbarton Oaks Papers, 72*, 25–48. https://doi.org/10.2307/26892563

Cumes, D. (2013). South African indigenous healing: How it works. *The Explorer, 9*(1), 58–65.

Dols, M. W. (1987). The origins of the Islamic hospital: Myth and reality. *Bulletin of the History of Medicine, 61*(3), 367–390.

Furniss, D. A. (1968). The monastic contribution to mediaeval medical care: Aspects of an earlier welfare state. *Journal of the Royal College of General Practitioners, 15*, 244–250.

Gilchrist, R. (2020). Spirit, mind and body: The archaeology of monastic healing. In *Sacred heritage: Monastic archaeology, material culture, and the body* (pp. 71–109). Cambridge University Press. https://doi.org/10.1017/9781108678087.004

Henderson, J. (2001). Healing the body and saving the soul: Hospitals in renaissance florence. *Renaissance Studies, 15*(2), 188–206.

Imhof, A. E. (1977). The hospital in the 18th century: For whom? The Charité Hospital in Berlin, the navy Hospital in Copenhagen, the Kongsberg Hospital in Norway. *Journal of Social History, 10*(4), 448–470. https://www.jstor.org/stable/3786763

Kolankaya-Bostanci, N. (2014). The evidence of shamanism rituals in early prehistoric periods of Europe and Anatolia. *Colloquium Anatolicum, 13*, 185–204.

Lankina, T., & Getachew, L. (2012). Mission or empire, word or sword? The human capital legacy in postcolonial democratic development. *American Journal of Political Science, 56*(2), 465–483. https://doi.org/10.1111/j.1540-5907.2011.00550.x

Lavigerie, C. (1874). Ordonnance au sujet de la direction des Séminaires 1874. In *Instructions aux missionnaires*, pp 250.

Levi, J. A. (2009). Portuguese and other European missionaries in Africa: A look at their linguistic production and attitudes (1415–1885). *Historiographia Linguistica, 36*(2/3), 363–392. https://doi.org/10.1075/hl.36.2-3.10lev

Maduro, R. (1983). Curanderismo and Latino views of disease and curing. *Western Journal of Medicine, 139*(6), 868–874.

Markham, J. G. (2010). *Ancient Babylonian medicine: Theory and practice*. Wiley-Blackwell.

Nunn, N. (2014). Gender and missionary influence in colonial Africa. In E. Akyeampong, R. H. Bates, N. Nunn, J. A. Robinson (Eds.), *Africa's development in historical perspective* (pp. 489–512). Cambridge University Press, Cambridge. https://doi.org/10.1017/CBO9781139644594.021

Pavli, A., & Maltezou, H. C. (2024). Asclepieia in ancient Greece: Pilgrimage and healing destinations, the forerunner of medical tourism. *Le Infezioni in Medicina, 32*(1), 113–115. https://doi.org/10.53854/liim-3201-15

Pawliková-Vilhanová, V. (2007). Christian missions in Africa and their role in the transformation of African societies. *Asian and African Studies 16,* (2), 249–260.

Price, N. S. (Ed.). (2001). *The archaeology of shamanism*. Routledge.

Riva, M. A., & Cesana, G. (2013). The charity and the care: The origin and the evolution of hospitals. *European Journal of Internal Medicine, 24*(1), 1–4. https://doi.org/10.1016/j.ejim.2012.11.002

Rosso, A. M. (2023). Methods and Management in Ancient Egyptian and Greek Medicine. *History and Philosophy of Medicine, 5*(3), 14. https://doi.org/10.53388/HPM2023014

Trotter, R. T., II. (1996). Curanderismo. In M. S. Micozzi (Ed.), *Fundamentals of complementary and alternative medicine* (1st ed., pp. 259–277). Churchill Livingstone.

Ethics at the Faith-Health Interface

1 Introduction

Public health is a *moral endeavor*, centered around the commitment to protect the vulnerable, alleviate suffering, and promote the flourishing of communities. Yet public health discourse often presents itself primarily in technical and administrative terms, obscuring the normative foundations that guide its decisions. The principles that justify prevention, regulation, and equity are not value-neutral; they reflect moral judgments about dignity, responsibility, and collective obligation. Making these ethical underpinnings explicit clarifies why religious traditions have historically resonated with public health commitments. While these aims are pursued through policies, for billions of people around the world, they are interpreted as spiritual mandates, whose recognition and leverage can improve trust, social cohesion, inclusion in public health initiatives, and emergency response capacity.

This chapter outlines the public health mandate and its ethical foundations, showing how core principles of as stewardship, dignity, solidarity, and care for the vulnerable are deeply embedded across religious traditions. It then examines how religious beliefs and practices understand health care as a sacred responsibility, and why faith-based organizations and leaders play a decisive role in trust, legitimacy, and community engagement. By illustrating the parallelism between public health ethics and religious doctrines, the chapter argues that religion can support public health professionals in building trust and connecting with the communities they serve. This perspective is reflected in collaborations promoted by the World Health Organization, which demonstrate how priorities such as vaccination, sanitation, and emergency preparedness can be framed as expressions of compassion, collective responsibility, and the sanctity of life (Winiger & Peng-Keller, 2021).

R. Bedi et al., *Faith Communities and Global Health*,
SpringerBriefs in Public Health, https://doi.org/10.1007/978-3-032-29417-3_2

2 Public Health

Public health is the science and art of promoting population health through collective, mainly preventive actions, in a manner that respects individuals' freedoms and minimizes health inequities (Coggon, 2023); thus, its goal is to maximize *public welfare* through policies that are population oriented and that regulate individual behavior. In this sense, the intrusion on individuals' autonomy must be (i) justified by the health gain generated by the policy; (ii) distributed to minimize inequalities across the broader population (Ng & Ruger, 2014).

The subject spans across government, business, and nonprofit sectors, whose decisions are guided by public health ethics principles. According to the American Public Health Association (2019), these consist of:

1) Professionalism and Trust—Public health practitioners must gain trust through a record of decisions based on evidence and the highest ethical, scientific, and professional standards.
2) Health and Safety—Public health practitioners and organizations have an ethical responsibility to prevent, minimize, and mitigate health harms
3) Health Justice and Equity—Public health practitioners must promote equitable distribution of burdens, benefits, and opportunities for health, reducing direct and indirect inequities.
4) Interdependence and Solidarity—Public health practitioners must recognize that the health of every individual depends on that of the members other ecosystems; thus, they must foster positive relationships among societies and environments.
5) Human Rights and Civil Liberties—Public health practitioners must respect personal autonomy, self-determination, and privacy.
6) Inclusivity and Engagement—Public health practitioners have the responsibility to include and engage diverse communities in their decision making.

Taken together, these principles articulate a coherent ethical system grounded in dignity, solidarity, and justice. Their language differs from theological doctrine, yet their normative structure parallels long-standing religious moral frameworks that likewise center the protection of vulnerable life and the regulation of communal conduct. Indeed, religious institutions commonly adopt codes of conduct for clergy and religious professionals, of which the Churches of England's pastor code is an example. These are based on explicit scriptural materials—e.g., Qur'anic and Prophetic teachings about trustworthiness—and serve to guide the behavior of religious leaders, whose role as both moral exemplars and practical guides of community life heavily depends on their perceived legitimacy.

Recognizing this structural convergence challenges the assumption that public health ethics are purely secular constructs detached from religious traditions.

The Parallel Between Public Health and Religion

Health and safety represent one of the clearest points of convergence between public health ethics and religious moral traditions. The link is strengthened by the faithful principle of stewardship, which recognizes believers as caretakers of what belongs to God—body, soul, community, environment—to whom they are accountable. As a result, in Judaism, the principle of *pikuach nefesh* establishes that *preventing danger* to life overrides all other religious commandments (*Muravsky* et al., 2021); this prioritization creates a strong theological basis for preventive measures aimed at reducing health risks. In Islam, the body is *amāna*, and individuals are morally accountable its protection and that of the others, which prohibits causing and reciprocating harm (Al Khayat, 2004).

Most faiths affirm that every life bears sacred worth, implying equal moral status before the Divine; this parallels the view that health is a fundamental human right, grounded in inherent *human dignity*, as articulated in the WHO Constitution's recognition of the highest attainable standard of health as a universal right (1948), and in the Universal Declaration of Human Rights' affirmation of equal dignity and the right to health and well-being (UN, 1948). Following this foundational thought, most religions understand inequalities as injustices and opposites to the principle of solidarity, which expresses the idea that human beings are bound together in moral community and share responsibility for one another's well-being. In Africa, Olivier et al. (2015) document that religious institutions provide a substantial share of healthcare services driven by the principle of solidarity.

Respect for individual dignity and moral agency constitutes a central ethical constraint on collective action in both public health and religious moral traditions. In Christianity, the moral limits placed on authority over the individual derive from the belief that each person bears inherent dignity as created in the image of God. Islamic ethics articulates a similarly structured but legally explicit approach to human rights and civil liberties. The Qur'an affirms the inherent dignity (*karāma*) of all human beings, while Islamic jurisprudence treats individuals as morally accountable agents responsible for their intentions and actions (Ghaly, 2013). At the same time, Islamic law recognizes that individual liberties may be constrained to protect public welfare (*maṣlaḥa*), particularly in contexts involving harm prevention. Crucially, such constraints are governed by established legal principles: necessity (*ḍarūra*) must be demonstrated, harm must be minimized, and restrictions must be proportionate and time-limited (Ghaly, 2013). Eventually, the procedural reasoning found in religious legal traditions—balancing necessity, proportionality, and collective welfare—mirrors the deliberative logic of modern public health regulation. This similarity complicates portrayals of secular governance as morally autonomous from religious thought, suggesting instead that both operate through structured ethical deliberation about risk, harm, and responsibility.

Despite the overlaps in the principles guiding public health and religious practice, Faith-Based Organizations (FBOs)'s engagement and inclusion in the former are limited by concerns of ideological conflict, misinformation, lack of literacy on specific contributions, as well as low availability of frameworks for effective engagement. This is especially detrimental to public health policies' design—which must be culturally sensitive—and adoption, as religions influence how individuals behave and view proposed public health interventions. The UNAIDS Framework for Partnership with Religious and Faith-Based Organizations (2009) documents that this is particularly true in sensitive domains such as vaccination, sexual and reproductive health, and end-of-life decision making (UNAIDS, 2009). For public health professionals, understanding these dynamics is essential to design effective, culturally respectful interventions (Koenig, 2012; Puchalski et al., 2009).

The Influence of Religion on Behavior

Rituals influence behavior at the daily and weekly level by normalizing embodied practices such as fasting, dietary regulation, hygiene, prayer, rest, and communal gathering. These routines shape attitudes toward the body, discipline, and self-care, and can either reinforce or complicate public health recommendations. For example, fasting can hinder medication adherence, while shared worship spaces can spread contagion. Rituals also structure behavior around calendar-based and life-event moments, including religious festivities, rites of passage, birth, and death. Periods such as religious holidays often involve intensified social interaction, which can increase health risks. These moments can function as barriers to care if misunderstood, or as opportunities for intervention when engaged respectfully.

Ethical frameworks complement ritual by guiding everyday decision making. These moral logics influence acceptance or refusal of interventions such as vaccination and reproductive health services.

How Religions Understand Health Care

Jewish tradition affirms medicine as a sacred endeavor rather than a secular intrusion. The Talmud recognizes healing as *mitzvah*, and the physician's role as a legitimate means through which life is preserved. This position is grounded in the principle of pikuach nefesh, which holds that preventing danger to life overrides nearly all other religious commandments. On this basis, Jewish legal reasoning has consistently supported preventive medical interventions *(Muravsky et al.*, 2021).

According to Muravsky et al. (2021), *halakhic* reasoning frames immunization as both a personal and communal responsibility to protect the vulnerable. While a minority dissent remains, often rooted in misinformation rather than doctrine, most rabbinic authorities affirm vaccination as a religious duty.

Islamic tradition likewise affirms medical treatment as religiously legitimate and ethically required. The Qur'an and Hadith recognize illness as part of human experience while affirming the permissibility of seeking medical treatment, with the prophetic teachings stating that for every disease, a cure exists. Healing (*shifāʾ*) is even one of God's names, highlighting medicine as participation in divine mercy. Islamic ethics grounds this position in established legal principles, particularly the prohibition of causing harm (*lā ḍarar wa-lā ḍirār*) and the obligation to protect public welfare (*maṣlaḥa*). Contemporary Islamic jurisprudence has applied this reasoning to modern preventive interventions, including vaccination and measures to control contagion (Al Khayat, 2004).

Christian ethics frames health care as a moral obligation grounded in the inherent dignity of every person and the duty to love one's neighbor. This ethic supports not only the treatment of the sick but also preventive action to protect others from harm. In contemporary Christian moral reasoning, public health interventions such as vaccination and infection control are widely regarded as ethically legitimate.

In Dharmic traditions, health care is justified through moral principles that underline the importance of achieving a state of harmony between body, mind, and spirit.

In Hinduism, medical treatment is supported by the principle of *dharma*, which frames care for the body and for others as part of right action that sustains social and moral order. Preventive and therapeutic practices, including long-standing medical systems such as Ayurveda, are integrated into everyday life and promoted through ethical self-discipline and service. Care for the sick is encouraged through *seva*, which frames caregiving as a moral duty within families, temples, and communities.

In Buddhism, medical treatment is legitimized through the ethical imperative to alleviate suffering (*dukkha*). Compassion (*karuṇā*) functions as a directive for action, supporting both treatment and prevention when these reduce harm to oneself and others. Care is promoted through monastic and lay practices that view of healing as a process of mindful awareness and ethical living.

In Sikhism, medical care and health-related service are explicitly promoted as expressions of religious commitment grounded in equality and *collective responsibility*. Principles of seva and the inherent dignity of all persons motivate organized community care, including food provision, medical aid, and disaster response. Care for health is treated as a shared obligation rather than individual charity, and while Sikhism does not operate through a formal legal code governing medical practice, community institutions actively promote and normalize care for the sick (Singh, 2022).

Across these traditions, health care is not conceptualized as a neutral technical service but as participation in moral order. Whether expressed through dharma, karuṇā, or seva, care for the body and protection of community are embedded within ethical systems that predate modern public health frameworks. This historical depth reinforces the potential for religious institutions to function as normative partners in health governance.

Recognizing the role of religious organizations and leaders in shaping trust, legitimacy, community participation, and equitable public health response, the WHO Guiding Principles (2021) establish engagement with religious leaders and faith communities as an ethical and operational necessity in health emergencies. The connection of public health and religious practice rests on the shared premise that every human life is valuable and must be protected through equitable access to care.

3 Conclusion

Together, the previous sections established that the relationship between public health and religion is not incidental but grounded in shared ethical commitments and lived social influence. Theological reflections offer a lens through which the moral nature of public health challenges becomes visible. Epidemics, environmental degradation, mental health crises, and population aging raise questions that exceed technical problem-solving and touch on suffering, responsibility, and the meaning of care. Faith traditions interpret epidemics as moments that test compassion and solidarity, shifting attention from causal blame to moral response. Environmental decline is understood, particularly within stewardship-based theologies, as a failure of humanity's obligation to protect God's creation. Mental illness exposes fractures in belonging, while aging and the end-of-life foreground dignity, accompaniment, and the sanctity of life. In these domains, theological perspectives do not replace scientific approaches but complement them by situating health within a broader account of humanity.

Ultimately, the convergence between public health ethics and religious moral reasoning underscores that health systems do not operate in ethically neutral environments. Their effectiveness depends not on technical design and normative legitimacy: where public health frameworks align with deeply embedded moral commitments, implementation gains traction, where they are perceived as detached from prevailing ethical systems, resistance may follow. Recognizing this dynamic reframes engagement with religious institutions as a structural consideration rather than a symbolic gesture.

At the same time, alignment between public health and religion is neither automatic nor free of tension. Historical and contemporary conflicts around vaccination, reproductive health, and evidence-based medicine illustrate how specific religious interpretations can clash with public health mandates. A mature engagement does not deny these tensions but treats them as sites for critical dialogue. Theology can interrogate its own traditions and correct harmful interpretations, while public health can remain attentive to questions of meaning, values, and trust.

References

Al Khayat, M. H. (2004). Health as a human right in Islam. World Health Organization, Regional Office for the Eastern Mediterranean. https://applications.emro.who.int/dsaf/dsa217.pdf.

American Public Health Association. (2019). *Public health code of ethics.*

Coggon, J. (2023). *What is public health?* Faculty of Public Health.

Ghaly, M. (2013). Islamic bioethics in the twenty-first century. *Zygon: Journal of Religion and Science*, *48*(3), 592–599. https://doi.org/10.1111/zygo.12021

Koenig, H. G. (2012). *Religion, spirituality, and health: the research and clinical implications.* ISRN Psychiatry: Article ID 278730. https://doi.org/10.5402/2012/278730

Muravsky, N. L., Betesh, G. M., McCoy, R. G. (2021). Religious doctrine and attitudes toward vaccination in Jewish Law. *Journal of Religion and Health, 62*(1), 373–388. https://pmc.ncbi.nlm.nih.gov/articles/PMC8549591/

Ng, N. Y., & Ruger, J. P. (2014). Ethics and social value judgments in public health. In A. J. Culyer (ed) *Encyclopedia of health economics* (vol. 1, pp. 287–291). Elsevier.

Olivier, J., Tsimpo, C., Renzaho, A., et al. (2015). Understanding the roles of faith-based health-care providers in Africa: Review of the evidence. *The Lancet, 386*(10005), 1765–1775. https://doi.org/10.1016/S0140-6736(15)60251-7

Puchalski, C., Ferrell, B., Virani, R., et al. (2009). Improving the quality of spiritual care as a dimension of palliative care: The report of the consensus conference. *Journal of Palliative Medicine, 12*(10), 885–904. https://doi.org/10.1089/jpm.2009.0142

Singh, S. P. (2022). Self and suffering in Indian thought: Implications for clinicians. *Bjpsych Advances, 28*(5), 286–296. https://doi.org/10.1192/bja.2022.1

UNAIDS. (2009). *Framework for partnership with religious and faith-based organisations.* https://www.unaids.org/sites/default/files/media_asset/20091201_framework_partnerships_en.pdf. Accessed 27 January 2026.

United Nations. (1948). *Universal declaration of human rights.* https://www.un.org/en/about-us/universal-declaration-of-human-rights. Accessed 28 January 2026.

Winiger, F., & Peng-Keller, S. (2021). Religion and the World Health Organization: An evolving relationship. *BMJ Global Health, 6*(4), e004073. https://gh.bmj.com/content/bmjgh/6/4/e004073.full.pdf

World Health Organization. (1948). *Constitution of the World Health Organization.* https://www.who.int/about/governance/constitution. Accessed 27 January 2026.

Faith-Based Health Systems Contribution

1 Introduction

Across low- and middle-income regions, *health gaps* are driven by various factors. In this context, faith-inspired institutions (FIIs) are long-standing components of the local health architecture and play a significant role in healthcare delivery, particularly where public systems are overwhelmed. Yet, their role is unevenly documented, and thus difficult to assess in a comparable manner across and within regions. Such uneven documentation shapes how faith-based actors are positioned marginally in policy frameworks, as well as their portrayal as peripheral actors despite structural integration within service delivery landscapes.

This section maps the contributions of faith-inspired institutions in providing healthcare services across low- and middle-income countries. By situating religious health networks within broader systems and highlighting the data gaps on their contributions, it clarifies the degree of both their embeddedness and exclusion. It reviews regional patterns of unmet health needs and constraints, summarizes available evidence on the institutional footprint of FIIs where data permit, and evaluates their role in healthcare provision, with the goal of clarifying where and how they complement public health systems under conditions of constrained capacity.

2 Sub-Saharan Africa

In the 2021 Universal Health Coverage (UHC) monitoring report, the score reached by the African region suggests that only a fraction of the healthcare needs of the population are being met with services of good quality and without an impoverishing effect on those who use them (Asamani et al., 2024). Indeed, every year an estimated 2.5 million avertable deaths occur in the area, of which almost 48% are due to poor quality of health care, while 52% are attributable to lack of access to health

R. Bedi et al., *Faith Communities and Global Health*,
SpringerBriefs in Public Health, https://doi.org/10.1007/978-3-032-29417-3_3

services (Kruk et al., 2018). Evidence from low-income countries further indicates that expanding healthcare coverage does not necessarily result in better outcomes, even for conditions highly amenable to medical care; rather, the quality of care seems to have a more decisive role in shaping health outcomes. As lower-income countries undergo epidemiological and demographic transitions, continued mortality reductions therefore depend not only on expanding coverage but on strengthening the quality of health systems alongside broader public health measures (Kruk et al., 2018).

Two of the key mechanisms through which deficits in quality persist are the quantitative shortfalls in the number of health workers and qualitative gaps in their competencies. The need-based requirement of health personnel is expected to increase by 21% between 2022 and 2030; of this need, only 49% will be met if the current trajectory of education outputs and training is maintained (Asamani et al., 2024). These constraints interact with other structural limitations, including inadequate infrastructure, equipment, and medical products, as well as improved public health programs, which further constrain the delivery of high-quality care.

At the same time, healthcare needs in the WHO African region are changing. According to the WHO (2025), the area is experiencing the persistence of infectious diseases alongside an increase in non-communicable diseases (NCDs), in the context of an aging population that is expected to reach 165 million people aged 60 years or older by 2050. Although access to care has almost doubled over the past twenty years, service delivery efforts have prioritized younger populations, leaving the needs for health and social care services of older adults largely unmet.

Given the limited availability of region-wide data on unmet health and social care needs among older populations, the WHO Research Report on Evidence Gaps on Unmet Health and Social Care Needs in the WHO African Region (WHO, 2025) uses Kenya as an illustrative case. In the 2018 Kenya Household Health Expenditure and Utilization Survey, 6.8% of the respondents were aged 60 years or older; among these, 37.8% reported a healthcare need during the four-week period prior to the survey, and 32% of those was unmet (WHO, 2025). Comparisons between participants with unmet and met healthcare needs show that unmet needs were less prevalent among urban residents and among wealthier and more educated groups, highlighting persistent socioeconomic inequities.

Market Shares of Faith-Inspired Healthcare Providers in SSA

Since the 1960s, estimates on the engagement of faith-inspired FIIs in healthcare provision have fallen in the 30% to 40% range in Sub-Saharan Africa, with substantial convergence across studies. However, these projections are likely to be inaccurate as (i) the absence of a widespread definition on FIIs hinders their coherent identification; (ii) the data on FIIs health service provision is measured across studies using diverse indicators and classifications, which hinder comparability, (iii) hospital services account for a small part of the overall health care provided (Olivier & Wodon, 2012).

Interpreting such approximations is especially difficult when one accounts for the fact that the total services included in these studies account for public and religious provision, leaving private contributions largely unexplored; this, despite the fact a large share of healthcare services is provided by actors outside the government.

All these factors are likely to contribute to an overestimation of the market share of FIIs in African national health systems. Evidence in this direction is represented by the results of Oliver and Wodon's (2012) review of household surveys on religious healthcare provision, whose estimates average around 6%. The 25% difference is largely explained by three elements. First, some households were unable to identify religious-based organizations. Second, in their answers, they considered the broader universe of health care, rather than hospitals alone. Third, while many of the countries considered in facility-based estimates are in conflict—and thus benefit from higher religious engagement—the sample of countries covered by the surveys is more balanced.

The divergence between facility-based and utilization-based estimates clarifies that the former captures the institutional footprint of faith-inspired institutions rather than their full contribution to healthcare delivery. This distinction is particularly salient given that many of their historical and ongoing contributions originate in community-based, preventive, and informal forms of care that remain weakly documented and largely uncaptured by standard health information systems. At the same time, high institutional presence should not be conflated with population reach or equity. Surely, the divergence across measures reveals how dominant measurement systems privilege certain forms of visibility while rendering others administratively secondary.

For these reasons, while policy claims based on a single metric are analytically fragile, facility-based evidence remains indispensable for understanding the structural role of FIIs within national health systems. The following section therefore adopts a facility-based mapping approach, not as a comprehensive measure of FII engagement, but as a means of situating their complementarities with public health systems.

Mapping Religious Contributions Across Uganda, Malawi, Zambia, Nigeria, and Tanzania

The Uganda Catholic Medical Bureau (UCMB) operates 296 Catholic health facilities, including 33 hospitals and 264 lower-level units. These account for 23% of Uganda's hospitals, and 27.5% of hospital bed capacity; they serve 15%–17% of the country's total population (UCMB, 2025). The Uganda Protestant Medical Bureau

(UPMB) manages 320-member health facilities, including 16 health training institutions with a significant rural presence, 10 Health Center IVs, 159 Health Center IIIs, 130 Health Center IIs, and 21 hospitals (UPMB, 2023).

In Malawi, the Christian Health Association of Malawi (CHAM) is the largest non-governmental health service provider, especially for remote and underserved areas. CHAM facilities provide around 30% of healthcare services, and train around 80% of medical professionals; the majority of these belongs to the Catholic Church (48%), followed by the Presbyterian Church (18%), the Anglican Church (11%), and the Seventh Day Adventist Church (10%) (KFW, 2023).

In Zambia, Catholic and Protestant Christian Missionary health workers formed the Churches Health Association of Zambia (CHAZ). The organization benefits from a fruitful relationship with the national Ministry of Health and oversees 152 institutions, including 36 hospitals, 84 rural health centers, and 32 community-based organizations (Zambia Ministry of Health & UNICEF, 2021). These account for 30% of Zambia's total healthcare facilities; the share raises above 50% in rural areas, reflecting the association's commitment to serving marginalized communities (Zambia Ministry of Health & UNICEF, 2021).

In Tanzania, the Christian Social Services Commission (CSSC) coordinates with Church health facilities falling under the Tanzanian Episcopal Conference and the Christian Council of Tanzania. These own 42% of hospitals and, in addition, offer pharmaceutical services and training via universities, colleges, and middle care training centers (CSSC, 2026). While no single nationwide Muslim health network exists, Muslim-affiliated organizations operate clinics and community health programs in the country. Reflecting Tanzania's religion diversity, the Tanzania Interfaith Partnership (TIP), set up in collaboration with UNICEF and UNFPA, developed a user-friendly violence prevention pocketbook to be distributed to more than 600 Christian and Muslim religious leaders. The pamphlet featured several religious writings condemning violence against women and children, encouraging positive gender norms and preventing violence (UNICEF, 2025).

In Nigeria, the Christian Health Association of Nigeria (CHAN) partners with government agencies at all levels and serves as the key coordinating body for a large network of church-run healthcare institutions—approximately 685 (CCIH, 2021). By contrast, Muslim faith-inspired healthcare provision follows a different institutional model: facilities are classified as private health facilities in national health databases; thus, they are dispersed across the health system. They account for over 10,000 facilities nationwide. Overall, faith-based health facilities provide primary, secondary, and tertiary healthcare services to 40% of Nigerians (CCIH, 2021).

The institutional asymmetry regarding the engagement of Muslim organizations has been partially offset through interfaith coordination mechanisms. In 2009, the Christian Interfaith Foundation for Public Health in Africa (CIFA)—an international faith-based organization working at the intersection of religion and health—supported the formation of the Nigerian Inter-Faith Action Association (NIFAA) in partnership with senior Muslim and Christian religious leaders. NIFAA was established to combat poverty and major communicable diseases and has worked closely with the National Malaria Control Program to train religious leaders to promote malaria prevention and treatment through sermons, community engagement, and faith-based messaging (Wise Solutions, 2011).

3 Eastern Mediterranean Region (EMRO)

In the Eastern Mediterranean Region, progress toward universal health coverage has been uneven; this has resulted in highly heterogeneous unmet healthcare needs, whose estimates range between around 10% in the Islamic Republic of Iran and 84% among Syrian refugees living in Lebanese camps (WHO, 2025).

The obstacles to effective healthcare provision can be analyzed at three different levels.

At the macro-level, armed conflict, *political instability*, displacement, and the COVID-19 pandemic have worsened health outcomes. Bouquet et al. (2021) report that mortality among patients with unsuccessful applications to exit the Gaza Strip to receive cancer treatment was significantly higher than mortality among patients whose permit was approved. In the Syrian Arab Republic, combat-related injuries have increased the burden on healthcare systems, while damage to hospitals has reduced healthcare capacity. Significant unmet healthcare needs have also been reported in externally displaced populations of refugees in the Islamic Republic of Iran, Jordan, and Lebanon because of barriers related to affordability and lack of access to healthcare services (WHO, 2025). At the meso-level, unmet needs are driven by inadequate infrastructure development, workforce shortages, insufficient training in geriatric and chronic care, and weaknesses in monitoring and improving service quality. At the micro-level, age, sex, income, education, and health literacy shape individuals' likelihood of experiencing unmet needs, with women, widows, and poorer households consistently more affected. The varied use of contributory systems across countries further exacerbates access to care; indeed, out-of-pocket expenditure in 2021 ranged from 6.1% in Oman to 77.2% in Afghanistan (WHO, 2025). Such costs disproportionately burden older people, especially given their lack of adequate income security.

Finally, *demographic trends* in the Eastern Mediterranean Region are expected to further increase the health gap. Indeed, while there have been some gains in life expectancy—with great variation also in this regard, as the population of Lebanon has experienced a 2.5 years rise, while that of Egypt has witnessed a 0.6-year loss (WHO, 2025)—these have not been mirrored by improved healthy life expectancy; this means that people will increasingly live in illness. Such evidence is even more worrying considering that among people aged 60 years or older, NCDs account for 1.8 million deaths out of 1.9; of these, over half are caused by cardiovascular diseases (WHO, 2025). Such trends will result in an increasing demand for long-term, integrated, and high-quality care that many health systems in the region are not yet equipped to deliver.

Market Shares of Faith-Inspired Healthcare Providers in EMRO

To date, the available evidence on the contribution of religious organizations to healthcare service provision in the WHO Eastern Mediterranean Region is characterized by severe *data limitations* that preclude system-level conclusions. There are no standardized, comparable estimates of the share of health care delivered by faith-inspired institutions across countries. This absence of systematic data does not imply the absence of institutional presence. Rather, it reflects limitations in reporting frameworks that frequently classify religious providers within broad private categories, obscuring their historical and operational distinctiveness. Even within countries, the literature reporting the engagement of FIIs in health is dominated by disease-specific, population-specific, or single country studies. This measurement gap undermines the incorporation of religious organizations into health system planning and financing frameworks and reinforces their marginalization in the humanitarian field.

Religious Contributions in Lebanon and Gaza

In Yemen, Islamic Relief operates in 13 of the country's governorates. The organization's programs cover the areas of emergency food assistance, food security, nutrition, health, water, sanitation and hygiene, orphan and child welfare. In 2022, Islamic Relief reached over 3.4 million people (Islamic Relief Worldwide, n.d.).

In Gaza, the Al-Ahli Hospital is the only Christian hospital in the Strip. During the conflict, its role has expanded dramatically to treat up to 750 patients per day, close to ten times its normal operating limit. Amid severe disruptions, forced evacuations of staff and patients, and damage to its infrastructure, the hospital continues to provide emergency and essential care (Anglican Overseas Aid, 2025).

Such cases illustrate that in fragile and conflict-affected settings, religious institutions often sustain service continuity when formal systems are destabilized. Their durability in crisis underscores the importance of recognizing religious infrastructures as components of resilience within health ecosystems.

4 South Asia

In South-East Asia, the negative correlation between the level of universal health coverage and out-of-pocket payments (OOPs) is stark; indeed, in countries where OOPs are extensively used (for example, in Bangladesh 74%, India 50.6%, and Myanmar 72.7%) the UHC service coverage index revolves around 50. Oppositely, in countries with low OOPs, like Thailand, the service coverage index rises to 80 (WHO, 2025).

Such differences across countries are reflected in the prevalence of unmet healthcare needs, whose estimations vary from 68.1% in Nepal to 1.5% in Thailand, with an average value of 18.3% (WHO, 2025). Yet, estimates are likely to underestimate the gap, given that most care in the region is provided by family members—and thus goes undetected—and formal, publicly funded social care systems are largely absent. A data analysis in Bangladesh shows that the main drivers of the care divide are the perception that health needs are not serious (21.4%), high *treatment costs* (68.0%), and distance to health facilities (4.9%) (WHO, 2025).

Today, more than 10% of the Region's population is over 60; this share is expected to triple by 2050, when the resulting increase in demand for health and social services will exacerbate current issues on health inequities and limited infrastructure (WHO, 2025).

Market Shares of Faith-Inspired Healthcare Providers in South Asia

Gathering data estimating the FIIs market share in South Asia is more challenging compared to Sub-Saharan Africa, where religious ownership of healthcare facilities is widely documented. This classification difficulty reflects a structural difference in how healthcare provision is organized across the region. Unlike parts of Sub-Saharan Africa, religious engagement in South Asia is frequently embedded within broader private, philanthropic, or community-based categories, rendering it less visible in formal mapping exercises while remaining socially influential.

The Christian Health Asset Mapping Consortium (CHAMC) reports that India hosts 815 Christian hospitals and 2434 Christian primary health facilities; in Indonesia, these numbers lower to 143 and 116, respectively (CHAMC, 2025). While large faith-linked networks are identified (e.g., Islamic Relief), no regional counts on hospitals, clinics, and beneficiaries are available for consultation; this largely reflects a different classification of healthcare provision and a more decentralized approach to it. Buddhist, Hindu, and Sikh interventions are institution specific.

Religious Contributions in India

In India, the Catholic Health Association of India (CHAI) operates through 11 regional units across the country; together, these manage 2345 health centers, 647 hospitals, and 35 nursing schools (CHAI, n.d.). Most of the care is delivered by full-time volunteers, mostly religious sisters belonging to different congregations. Key areas of intervention are community health, maternal and child health, rehabilitation and disaster relief (CHAI, n.d.).

Sikh interventions are often highly visible in crisis response and community support. For example, Khalsa Aid—an international humanitarian relief organization rooted in Sikh principles and operating as a nonprofit organization—played a significant role in India's COVID-19 relief efforts by distributing essential supplies to affected communities and delivering oxygen concentrators and medical equipment via the Dharma Bharathi Mission (Khalsa Aid, n.d.).

Hindu interventions can be distinguished between those financing healthcare interventions and those supporting culturally embedded healing practices. Among the former, the Sri Venkateswara Pranadana Trust aims to provide free medical care to poor patients afflicted by chronic, life-threatening conditions via the hospitals run by the Tirumala Tirupati Devasthanams (Tirumala Tirupati Devasthanams, n.d.). Among the latter, the Patanjali Yogpeeth (Haridwar) aims to increase the propagation of yoga and Ayurveda via classes, courses, and research as methods of health promotion and healing (Telles et al., 2013). Buddhist interventions mainly assume a philanthropic note.

The diversity of organizational forms across South Asia reflects plural models of religiously informed care, rather than a unified infrastructural template.

5 Latin America

In 2019, the UHC score of Latin America fell in the 50–79 range; this variation was reflected in that of unmet healthcare needs, which spanned from around 10% in Chile (2022) to around 72% in Peru (PAHO, 2024)—with an overall stable reporting population across years. During the COVID-19 pandemic, all countries with available data experienced an increase in unmet healthcare needs; the average jump was around 20% and was particularly high among the poorest quintiles, who already faced the highest rates of foregone care (PAHO, 2024).

The causes of the health gap are multifaceted and comprise *organizational barriers* (21.5%), financial barriers (14.2%), availability issues, acceptability issues, and geographic barriers; the importance of each obstacle varies by country, with financial barriers assuming a minimal role in El Salvador (2022) and a prevalent one in Honduras (2019) (PAHO, 2024). In 2019, between 1.5% and 7.8% of the overall population faced catastrophic health expenses. Rural households consistently faced greater exposure than urban households; for example, in Peru, 48.9% of rural households experienced impoverishment due to health costs, compared with 13.1% of urban households (PAHO, 2024).

These differentiated barriers create spaces in which faith-based actors may intervene not solely through institutional ownership of facilities, but through localized networks of solidarity and outreach. In several countries, religious organizations function as intermediaries between vulnerable populations and formal health systems, particularly where public trust or administrative reach is uneven.

Alongside these coverage and access gaps, Latin America is undergoing a pronounced *demographic* and *epidemiologic transition*. Declining fertility and increasing life expectancy have led to rapid population aging, shifting the disease burden away from infectious causes toward chronic non-communicable diseases and increasing demand for long-term, continuous care. Consequently, deaths from non-communicable diseases, such as cardiovascular diseases, cancer, and diabetes, increased 43% in the Americas region since 2000, reaching six million in 2021. According to the report Las ENT de un vistazo 2025, cardiovascular diseases lead the way, followed by cancer, diabetes, and chronic respiratory diseases (WHO, 2025). Eventually, such prevalence is exacerbated by high obesity rates and environmental challenges.

Market Shares of Faith-Inspired Healthcare Providers in Latin America

In Latin America, the contribution of faith-based organizations to healthcare delivery cannot be systematically quantified due to the lack of comparable regional or country level data. Health information systems and household surveys in the region do not identify providers by religious affiliation, and faith-based facilities are subsumed within broad private nonprofit categories. In addition, faith-based health provision in Latin America is fragmented and largely lacks national umbrella organizations.

Religious Contributions in Brazil

In Brazil, the organization Pastoral da Criança significantly contributed to the reduction of infant and maternal mortality rates in the country. Today, they are expanding their mission to cover nutrition-related health needs (Pastoral da Criança, n.d.).

6 Global Faith-Based Networks and Collaborations

At the global level, several international coalitions provide platforms for faith-health engagement. These coalitions reflect a level of institutional consolidation that extends beyond localized service provision. They demonstrate that faith-based engagement in health operates within transnational governance spaces, interfacing directly with multilateral organizations and national ministries rather than functioning solely at community level.

The World Council of Churches (WCC) is a global fellowship of Christian churches that work together for unity, justice, and peace mainly via advocacy efforts. Indeed, the WCC functions primarily as a convening body leveraging its role as a fellowship of churches to shape ethical frameworks and engage multilaterally, including with WHO and the UN (WCC, n.d.). Caritas Internationalis—a global confederation of Catholic organizations—by contrast, is an operational confederation rooted in the Catholic Church, distinguished by its extensive national-level presence through diocesan Caritas organizations that deliver health, social protection, and humanitarian services directly to communities, often embedded within public welfare systems (Caritas Internationalis, n.d.).

ACT Alliance adds value through coordination and surge capacity: as a coalition of Protestant and Orthodox agencies, it specializes in joint humanitarian response, pooled funding, and collective advocacy, enabling members to scale health and emergency interventions (ACT Alliance, n.d.). Finally, World Vision International is a Christian humanitarian organization dedicated to working with children, families, and communities to overcome poverty and injustice (World Vision International, n.d.). It is characterized by its long-term, area-based development model, combining health, child protection, and livelihoods within multi-year community partnerships, with a strong emphasis on monitoring outcomes for children (World Vision International, n.d.).

Among global Islamic faith-based organizations, Islamic Relief Worldwide is a humanitarian and development organization operating in response to emergencies and chronic poverty, with a strong emphasis on health, nutrition, livelihoods, and social protection, delivered through country offices and partnerships in conflict-affected and fragile settings (Islamic Relief Worldwide, n.d.). The Aga Khan Development Network (AKDN), instead, consists of a group of private agencies working across health, education, social protection, and economic development, with a major added value in institutional service delivery, including hospitals, clinics, and health professional training institutions integrated into national health systems, particularly in low-income and pluralistic contexts (AKDN, n.d.). Muslim Aid provides development support via partnership with local organizations and community empowerment, rather than large institutional health systems (Muslim Aid, n.d.). Finally, the International Islamic Relief Organization (IIRO), affiliated with the Muslim World League, emphasizes charitable, humanitarian, and relief activities rooted in Islamic solidarity, with a particular focus on emergency assistance, health support, social care, and aid delivery.

Among global Buddhist relief organizations, the Tzu Chi Foundation is known for implementing large-scale disaster relief, medical and community health programs, all grounded in Buddhist principles of charity and volunteer service (Tzi Chi Foundation, n.d.). Oppositely, the International Buddhist Relief Organization (IBRO) focuses on supporting vulnerable populations through community-driven projects that reflect Buddhist teachings on alleviating suffering; it emphasizes collaboration among Buddhist communities to respond to crises and long-term needs. Finally, the Buddhist Global Relief (BGR) organization concentrates on hunger relief and food security, partnering with local organizations globally to implement feeding programs, agricultural support, and nutrition initiatives, explicitly linking these efforts to Buddhist principles of right livelihood and compassion for the hungry (Buddhist Global Relief, n.d.).

Within Hindu and Sikh faith-based networks, the Ramakrishna Mission is a monastic organization providing institutional health service delivery (Belur Math-Ramakrishna Mission, n.d.). The Chinmaya Mission positions its contribution primarily through preventive health, mental well-being, and values-based education, rather than large-scale clinical provision; its health-related work focuses on yoga, stress management, counselling, and holistic well-being programs delivered through centers, camps, and educational institutions (Chinmaya Mission, n.d.).

Evaluation of the Provision of Healthcare Services by Faith-Inspired Institutions

From a service-provision perspective, faith-inspired healthcare providers present several operational strengths. Their embedded presence within communities enables early identification of underserved populations and facilitates service delivery to groups that are often poorly reached by public or for-profit providers. Where mapping of religious contribution exists (e.g., in the African continent), its social penetration supports partnerships with public authorities, allowing coordinated interventions. Faith-based providers access to volunteer networks can partially mitigate workforce shortages, provided that volunteers receive appropriate training and supervision; their faith-based ethics support resilience in crisis settings.

At the same time, significant limitations remain. In many contexts, the absence of comprehensive mapping and reporting hinders partnerships and perpetuates inefficiencies, both among faith-based providers themselves and between them and the public sector. The evidence gap also obstacles financial integration with public health systems, which limits predictable funding flows and continuity in operations in faith-run facilities. This exacerbates the precariousness of relying on volunteers, which also raises questions about quality of care where training standards differ from those applied to salaried health professionals.

Service delivery may also be fragmented, with providers offering stand-alone services that are poorly integrated national healthcare systems; this is especially true where service provision is concentrated in specific geographic and clinical areas.

7 Conclusion

This chapter has shown that FIIs offer a substantial share of institutional health service and play a complementary role in extending service availability, especially in rural and underserved areas. Their embedded community presence, capacity to mobilize volunteers, and operational resilience during crises allow them to reach populations that are often missed by public and for-profit providers.

At the same time, the analysis highlights persistent constraints that limit their integration in broader health systems. Overall, the contributions of FIIs are context specific and vary based on the degree of institutional integration. Strengthening the role of FIIs within health systems therefore requires moving beyond broad claims about market share, toward improved mapping, routine reporting, and structured partnerships that align service delivery with national health priorities.

References

ACT Alliance. (n.d.). About Us. https://actalliance.org/about-us/. Accessed 01 August 2025

Aga Khan Development Network. (n.d.). *Who we are.* https://the.akdn/en/who-we-are. Accessed August 5, 2025.

Anglican Overseas Aid. (2025). *Ahli Arab Hospital—Church update.* https://anglicanoverseasaid.org.au/our-work/disaster-response/ahli-arab-hospital/. Accessed July 27, 2025.

Asamani, J. A., Bediakon, K. S. B., Boniol, M., Munga'tu, J. K., Akugri, F. A., Muvango, L. L., Bayiga, E. D. Z., Christmals, C. D., Okoroafor, S., Titus, M. & Titi-Ofei, R. (2024). Projected health workforce requirements and shortage for addressing the disease burden in the WHO Africa Region, 2022–2030: A needs-based modeling study. *BMJ Global Health, 7,* e015972. https://doi.org/10.1136/bmjgh-2024-015972.

Belur Math-Ramakrishna Mission. (n.d.). Service—Medical. https://belurmath.org/. Accessed July 29, 2025.

Bouquet, B., Barone-Adesi, F., Lafi, M., et al. (2021). Comparative survival of cancer patients requiring Israeli permits to exit the Gaza Strip for health care: A retrospective cohort study from 2008 to 2017. *PLoS ONE, 16*(6), Article e0251058. https://doi.org/10.1371/journal.pone.0251058

Buddhist Global Relief. (n.d.). Current Projects. https://buddhistglobalrelief.org/current-projects/. Accessed August 5, 2025.

Caritas Internationalis. (n.d.). *Who we are.* https://www.caritas.org/who-we-are/. Accessed August 10, 2025.

Catholic Health Association of India. (n.d.). What we do. https://chai-india.org/association_what-we-do/. Accessed February 9, 2026.

Chinmaya Mission. (n.d.). *The mission.* https://www.chinmayamission.com/global/themission. Accessed August 20, 2025.

Christian Connections for International Health. (2021). *An overview of the health system in Nigeria and the contributions and role of faith-based health providers in the overall health system.* https://www.ccih.org/wp. Accessed July 23, 2025.

Christian Health Asset Mapping Consortium. (2025). *Initial data brief on Christian health assets in 11 Asian Countries.* Washington, DC. https://faithhealthassets.org/. Accessed July 27, 2025.

Christian Social Services Commission. (2026). *Health services.* https://cssc.or.tz/our-work/health-services. Accessed August 10, 2025.

Islamic Relief Worldwide. (2023). *Islamic Relief Yemen annual report 2022.* London. https://islamic-relief.org/wp-content/uploads/2023/09/IRYemen-AR2022.pdf. Accessed July 25, 2025.

Islamic Relief Worldwide. (n.d.). *About us.* https://islamic-relief.org/about-us/. Accessed August 5, 2025.

Khalsa Aid. (2021). *COVID-19 relief in India.* https://khalsaaid.org/projects/india/2021/covid-19-relief-in-india. Accessed 9 February 2026

KfW Development Bank. (2023). *Ex-post evaluation: Strengthening public-private partnerships in the health sector, Malawi.* https://www.bmz.de/en. Accessed 20 July 2025

Khalsa Aid. (2021). *COVID-19 relief in India*. https://khalsaaid.org/projects/india/2021/covid-19-relief-in-india. Accessed February 9, 2026.

Kruk, M. E., Gage, A. D., Joseph, N. T., et al. (2018). Mortality due to low-quality health systems in the universal health coverage era: A systematic analysis of amenable deaths in 137 countries. *The Lancet, 392*(10160), 2203–2212. https://doi.org/10.1016/S0140-6736(18)31668-4

Muslim Aid. (n.d.). *About us*. https://www.muslimaid.org/about-us/. Accessed August 10, 2025.

Olivier, J., & Wodon, Q. (2012). Faith-inspired health care providers in sub-Saharan Africa and public-private partnerships: A brief overview. In Olivier & Wodon (ed). *The role of faith-inspired health care providers in Sub-Saharan Africa and public-private partnerships: Strengthening the evidence for faith-inspired health engagement in Africa. (HNP) Discussion Paper* (Vol. 1, pp. 11–26). World Bank.

Pan American Health Organization. (2024). *Progress in universal health in the Americas: Addressing unmet healthcare needs, gaps in coverage, and lack of financial protection, through primary health care*. https://doi.org/10.37774/9789275129470.

Pastoral da Criança. (2026). *Pastoral da Criança celebrates 30 years of social action for the reduction of infant mortality*. https://www.pastoraldacrianca.org.br/en/news/2777. Accessed February 13, 2026.

Telles, S., Yadav, A., Bhardwaj, A. K., Sharma, S. K., & Singh, N. (2013). Patanjali Yogpeeth, Haridwar: An Ayurveda center which includes treatment, research, and education. *Journal of Ayurveda and integrative Medicine, 4*, 120–2. https://doi.org/10.4103/0975-9476.113885.

Tirumala Tirupati Devasthanams. "Sri Venkateswara Pranadana Trust." Tirumala Tirupati Devasthanams. https://www.tirumala.org/SriVenkateswaraPranadanaTrust.aspx. Accessed February 9, 2026.

Tzu Chi Foundation. (n.d.). *Charity: We do—Charity*. https://global.tzuchi.org/we-do_charity. Accessed August 5, 2025.

Uganda Catholic Medical Bureau. (2025). *History*. https://www.ucmb.co.ug/history/. Accessed July 20, 2025.

Uganda Protestant Medical Bureau. (2023). *Uganda protestant medical bureau annual report 2022–2023: Preferred Christian health care partner for sustainable services*. https://upmb.co.ug/wp-content/uploads/2024/05/. Accessed July 20, 2025.

UNICEF Tanzania. (2025). *Preventing violence through religion*. https://www.unicef.org/tanzania/stories/preventing-violence-through-religion. Accessed August 20, 2025.

Wise Solutions, L. L. C. (2011). *Faiths United for Health Campaign: Evaluation report*. Wise Solutions, LLC.

World Council of Churches. (n.d.). *About the WCC*. https://www.oikoumene.org/about-the-wcc. Accessed August 5, 2025.

World Health Organization. (2025). *Evidence gaps on unmet health and social care needs in the WHO African region: Research report*. Monitoring Universal Health Coverage in Ageing Populations. World Health Organization. https://iris.who.int/.

World Health Organization. (2025). *Evidence gaps on unmet health and social care needs in the WHO Eastern Mediterranean Region: Research Report*. Monitoring Universal Health Coverage in Ageing Populations. World Health Organization. https://iris.who.int/.

World Health Organization. (2025). *Evidence gaps on unmet health and social care needs in the WHO South-East Asia Region: Research Report*. World Health Organization, Centre for Health Development (WHO Kobe Centre). https://wkc.who.int/.

World Health Organization. Noncommunicable Diseases in the Americas: Las ENT de un vistazo 2025. Washington, DC: Pan American Health Organization/World Health Organization, 2025. Accessed February 9, 2026. https://iris.paho.org/items/9fdcb9d5-89fb-4906-bacd-62a0d051f122.

World Vision International. (n.d.). *About us*. https://www.wvi.org/about-us. Accessed August 5, 2025.

Zambia Ministry of Health and UNICEF. (2021). *National community health strategy operational plan*. https://www.unicef.org/zambia/media/5796/file/MOH. Accessed July 20, 2025.

Faith and Trust in Health Crises

1 Introduction

Health emergencies disrupt not only health systems but also shared frameworks of meaning. In such moments, responses to diseases are shaped both by the availability of medical interventions and by the way communities interpret and accept them.

This section examines the role of religious leadership during Ebola, HIV/AIDS, and COVID-19, focusing on how faith mediated trust, compliance, and care at the community level. Rather than assessing institutional performance, it analyzes how religious narratives and practices shaped lived responses to public health measures.

By comparing these cases across different temporal and epidemiological contexts, we show that the influence of faith depends on institutional engagement and timing. The comparison also highlights how historical memory—particularly experiences of colonial medical intervention and external control—continues to influence contemporary responses to health authority. Understanding faith engagement therefore requires situating emergency response within longer trajectories of trust, power, and institutional recognition. Studying these dynamics is necessary to understand why similar public health strategies produce divergent social responses, and why effective emergency response requires attention to meaning.

2 Faith Leadership in Time of Emergencies

In the period 249–262 CE, the Plague of Cyprian ravaged the Roman Empire. In this context, Christians refused to abandon the afflicted; they nursed the sick, provided food, and buried the dead, while pagan neighbors often fled or neglected the dying (Pamphilus, 1703). Confirming this, Dionysius of Alexandria praised Christians' unbounded care for the sick while he condemned pagans for abandoning the ill (Hoeldtke, 2021).

R. Bedi et al., *Faith Communities and Global Health*,
SpringerBriefs in Public Health, https://doi.org/10.1007/978-3-032-29417-3_4

In the following centuries, numerous plague outbreaks spread across Europe. After the Plague of Justinian (541–543 CE) and the Black Death (1347–1351), *Yersinia pestis* emerged in recurrent waves throughout the early modern period (Piret & Boivin, 2021). One of the most severe of these outbreaks was the plague of Milan in 1630. In this context, the physician Abraham Catalano documented how Christian and Jewish communities adapted religious life under epidemic restrictions, including conducting worship from domestic windows, within formally regulated urban ghettos (Waxman, 2020).

These accounts illustrate long-standing cases of religious care during epidemics and precede the emergence of formal health systems; more recent interventions therefore offer clearer insight into how religious actors interact with public health institutions in crisis settings.

Ebola Epidemic in West Africa

The 2014–2016 Ebola outbreak was the largest and most devastating since the virus was first discovered, affecting primarily Guinea, Liberia, and Sierra Leone and spreading to Nigeria, Senegal, Mali, Spain, the United Kingdom, and the United States (WHO, n.d.). Whereas earlier Ebola outbreaks occurred in relatively isolated areas and followed a recurring pattern of local containment, the West African epidemic unfolded in a context shaped by decades of political instability, cross-border mobility, and fragile health infrastructures, transforming a previously sporadic disease into a prolonged international emergency.

The first confirmed case of Ebola was officially reported by the Guinea Ministry of Health on March 23, 2014 (Dixon & Schafer, 2014). In response, national ministries of health, with the support of Médecins Sans Frontières (MSF) and WHO, began establishing Ebola Treatment Centres (ETCs) in affected regions. However, the absence of robust disease surveillance systems significantly hindered early containment efforts. To strengthen the response, teams from the US Centers for Disease Control and Prevention (CDC) were deployed under the Global Outbreak Alert and Response Network (GOARN), providing technical assistance in case investigation, contact tracing, and data collection to support national control strategies.

Governments enforced quarantines, curfews, border controls, and travel restrictions, which while essential for containment, also posed difficulties due to the poverty of isolated communities by cutting off subsistence livelihoods, disrupting food access, and imposing isolation without adequate support. Consequently, the most fragile populations relied on World Food Program efforts to fight starvation (O'Carroll, 2014).

As local systems became overwhelmed, virus transmission in healthcare facilities and deaths among healthcare workers begun, resulting in the overall collapse of the healthcare system (Dixon & Schafer, 2014). By June 2014, the disease fatality rate across all infected countries was 64% (Dixon & Schafer, 2014).

In this situation, international organizations, including WHO, MSF, CDC and UNICEF, stepped in with treatment, outreach, and logistics support. Initially, the response was slow and complicated for numerous reasons, including wide geographic spread of cases, population mobility, poor public health infrastructure, local unfamiliarity with Ebola, and distrust of health workers and governments (Bell et al., 2016). Mistrust was amplified by rumors that pictured Ebola as a Western agenda, reinforcing resistance toward response teams.

In this context, religious leaders and faith-based organizations (FBOs) emerged as critical partners to alleviate concerns of hesitant populations, as well as to bridge the gap between public health messaging and local communities.

Cultural Blind Spots in Ebola Containment

At the beginning of the outbreak in Guinea, a pregnant woman died with what was suspected to be a severe Ebola infection. Medical authorities encouraged a safe burial rite to avoid contagion; however, the community feared the deviance from traditional burial rituals would result in a curse that might descend upon the woman's village. Indeed, the local understanding of death involves resolving challenges that emerged between family and expressing affection through body contact to help the death move with ease into the afterlife. If the correct funeral procedures aren't followed, the community may be judged "at fault" by the ancestors, who might levy a curse on the group. The family and village prioritized compliance with spiritual traditions over public health regulations; consequently, they insisted on performing the caesarean and refused to provide a list of the deceased woman's contacts for tracing (Anoko & Henry, 2020). Eventually, this confrontation exposes a disconnect between externally imposed protocols and locally embedded systems of meaning.

Overall, the top-down imposition of funeral procedures to contain infection by government officials, who were deeply mistrusted by local communities, resulted in families hiding infected people or conducting secret burials, which perpetuated transmission (Marshall, 2016). Such imposition reinforced historical memories of externally directed medical interventions, amplifying suspicions that public health measures served interests beyond community welfare. In this context, *mistrust* was rooted in longer trajectories of unequal medical governance. The fact that figures with moral authority as imams and pastors weren't involved further expanded the idea that outsiders were disrespecting the death (Marshall, 2016). Finally, communications were delivered through technical language focused on the deadliness of the disease, without any adaptation to local beliefs—which believed the disease to be caused by spiritual imbalance.

The Mobilization of Religious Networks in Crisis

The penetration of FBOs in the healthcare system helped public authorities get compliance rather than resistance from local communities. For example, in several

Liberian settings, collaborative messaging from both governmental and religious authorities helped facilitate voluntary adherence to public health quarantine protocols, suggesting that co-produced public messaging had a persuasive effect on behavioral change (Arthur et al., 2023).

Despite their potential in improving effectiveness of health interventions, religious leaders were not meaningfully engaged in the initial phases of the Ebola response. International responders worked almost exclusively through state and humanitarian institutions, and religious practices were treated as sources of risk rather than as sites for negotiated change (Marshall, 2016). Active collaboration only began in late 2014, by which time it had become clear that medical containment strategies were insufficient on their own due to their inability to persuade resistant communities.

By leveraging their authority, Christian and Muslim leaders influenced communities into accepting life-saving advice from health workers, offered *religious context* to new burial practices, and reduced violence directed at response teams. Communities that had rejected official directives began to comply with them; as a result, infection rates declined, and health interventions reached previously resistant areas (Bedson et al, 2020).

The Origins of Mistrust and the Role of Religion

Before colonialism, Traditional Medicine (TM), defined as the sum of the knowledge, skills, and practices based on the theories, beliefs, and experiences indigenous to different cultures used in the maintenance of health, as well as in the prevention, diagnosis, and treatment of illnesses (WHO, 2000), used to be the dominant medical system in much of Saharan Africa, South Asia, and Indigenous Americas. TM would be implemented by traditional doctors, who attempted to reconnect the social and emotional equilibrium of patients based on community relationships (Hillenbrand, 2006 in Abdullahi, 2011).

Colonialism contributed to the stigmatization of TM, which was viewed by Western countries as a form of witchcraft and thus backwardness (Abdullahi, 2011). Often, this practice was delegated to churches, which reinforced their presence as holders of local traditions and identity (Amster, 2022). Christian symbolism, for example, aligned with African traditional therapeutic systems, through practices as blessing the sick, prayers, and social support. Especially in the early colonial phase, religious organizations influenced local communities and posed themselves as providers of care.

In several colonial settings, health interventions were implemented by external authorities with limited attention to consent, explanation, or follow-up. For example, French colonial governments undertook extensive medical campaigns against sleeping sickness in SSA through forced medication, which would sometimes result in blindness and death (Lowes & Montenero, 2021).

Lowes and Montero (2021) state that being forcibly examined and injected fed deep-seated mistrust among Africans toward Western medicine. This feeling was reinforced by the understanding that receiving health care would benefit Western interests; indeed, in a colonial healthcare system, colonizers are directed toward well-funded, modern hospitals, while the colonized receive cure with the purpose of preserving their productivity in the labor force and/or preventing revolution, and are thus treated in inferior hospitals (Amster, 2022). Eventually, colonial practices in the medical field were referred to by The Lancet as a form of new imperialism (The Lancet, 2004).

In the age of decolonization, politicians promised independence would enable the removal of the health inequities that had characterized the colonial rule, by restoring national control over health priorities. In practice, however, post-independence healthcare expansion often relied on externally financed, vertically organized programs that reproduced top-down decision making and limited community participation. Investment remained concentrated in urban centers that had served as colonial administrative hubs, reinforcing long-standing rural–urban disparities and perpetuating unequal access to care.

The HIV/AIDS Emergency

During the early years of the HIV/AIDS pandemic, particularly throughout the 1980s and 1990s, HIV spread rapidly across Sub-Saharan Africa due to a combination of viral dynamics, population vulnerability, and systemic weaknesses. These consisted in the presence of vulnerable groups—including sex workers and displaced populations—the insufficient health infrastructure, the limited public awareness, and low education levels. As a consequence, prevalence across SSA increased from 6.74% in 1990 to 9.04% in 1994 (Adams et al., 2023), becoming a major public health epidemic.

In the 1980s, the role of churches was ambivalent, and care coexisted with silence or *moral condemnation*. On the one hand, many religious leaders viewed HIV as a divine punishment for moral transgressions such as promiscuity and homosexuality (Kruger et al., 2025). Eventually, such interpretations drew on long-standing theological traditions linking illness to moral disorder, which aligned with the early concentration of HIV among stigmatized groups. As a result, interpretations in parts of Sub-Saharan Africa emphasized faith as a sufficient treatment to HIV/AIDS (Azia et al., 2023). On the other hand, churches took care of infected people by opening their mission hospitals to patients and assisting orphaned children.

It was only between 1990 and 2010, after realizing religious groups were not immune to HIV, that organizations began to re-evaluate their role in epidemic management. Gradually, churches and mosques recognized social stigma as one of the most damaging consequences of the disease—and acknowledged their own role in perpetuating it.

The lack of coordination among Catholic HIV responses prompted the Southern African Catholic Bishops' Conference (SACBC), in partnership with the Catholic Medical Mission Board (CMMB), to launch the Choose to Care initiative in 2000 (Krüger, 2009). Initially focused on prevention and care, the program later expanded to support treatment access for orphans and vulnerable children, working alongside government efforts (UNAIDS, 2006). For some Pentecostal Christians, ART was understood as consistent with divine providence—for example, as knowledge given by God to scientists—thereby supporting adherence (Azia et al., 2023).

In 2002, Rev. Canon Gideon Byamugisha, the first African religious leader to publicly disclose his HIV-positive status, founded the African Network of Religious Leaders Living with or Personally Affected by HIV and AIDS (ARENELA +). Operating initially in East and Southern Africa and later expanding globally as INERELA + , the network currently works through interfaith clergy platforms to reduce HIV-related stigma by promoting public disclosure, reshaping theological narratives, and integrating faith actors into national and international HIV responses (IRENELA + , n.d.).

By 2010s, the scale-up of antiretroviral therapy transformed HIV into a chronic condition requiring community support and stigma reduction. Governments and international donors recognized that faith-based actors were already providing support and reducing stigma on the ground; thus, SACBC partnered with the German Catholic agency Misereor to expand treatment access to through the AIDS Data System (ADS), a real-time platform used to monitor patients and link them to care. In 2015, during the United Nations General Assembly, UNAIDS and PEPFAR launched a two-year, four million US dollar initiative to strengthen FBO-led HIV service delivery, marking the large-scale inclusion of FBOs within global HIV policy frameworks (UNAIDS, 2015, 2020).

HIV in Uganda. In Uganda, where urban HIV prevalence approached 30% in 1990 (Uganda AIDS Commission, 2023)—among the highest globally—the crisis was exacerbated by the country's fragile healthcare system.

Recognizing the urgency of the epidemic and the state's weakness, President Yoweri Museveni, pragmatically endorsed a government-led public health campaign that involved training, education, and communication strategies under the banner of "Abstinence, Be faithful and, if necessary, use Condoms." The initiative heavily relied on the mobilization of community leaders and religious institutions, which emphasized the "A" and "B" components—encouraging young people to abstain from sex before marriage and urging spouses to remain faithful. Within many churches and mosques, the "C" was often reframed as a call for character formation, promoting discipline and marital fidelity rather than condom distribution.

The alignment between public policy and pulpit messaging helped build community trust and cultural legitimacy around HIV prevention efforts. Eventually, Uganda saw a remarkable decline in infection rates, which dropped to 8% by 2002 (Bunson, 2008). According to the Demographic and Health Survey, 93% of Ugandans reported having altered their sexual behavior to avoid contracting HIV/AIDS (Bunson, 2008).

Soon, this behavioral foundation expanded into more institutional responses: organizations like the Uganda Joint Christian Council and the Islamic Medical Association of Uganda took the lead in promoting HIV testing, supporting antiretroviral treatment, and establishing homes for HIV orphans.

The COVID-19 Pandemic

The COVID-19 pandemic emerged at the end of 2019, following an outbreak of atypical pneumonia in Wuhan, China. By January 5, 2020, the WHO had issued its first Disease Outbreak News, triggering the activation of an Incident Management Support Team. Over the following weeks, confirmed human-to-human transmission and rapid geographic spread intensified global concerns: by January 13, the first case outside China was reported in Thailand; in the following days, cases had been confirmed in Japan, South Korea, and the United States. Daily reported cases rose sharply; in this context of accelerating transmission, the outbreak was declared a Public Health Emergency of International Concern on January 30, before being classified as a global pandemic in mid-March 2020 (WHO, 2020). As of December 2023, over 772 million confirmed cases and nearly 7 million deaths had been reported globally (WHO, 2023).

Since January 2020, governments around the world implemented sweeping public health measures, including travel restrictions, social distancing mandates, lockdowns, mask requirements, and vaccine rollouts. Vaccine uptake, however, was uneven across regions. In parts of Europe, Russia, and the Middle East, misinformation, disinformation, and concerns about vaccine safety fueled skepticism despite rapid vaccine development. In Africa, low vaccination coverage reflected a combination of delayed and limited access, as well as vaccine hesitancy. As a result, by 2021 around 59% of Europe's population was vaccinated, while the vaccination uptake rate in Africa was around 8% (Armstrong, 2021).

Building on Ebola and HIV experiences about the role of faith institutions in transmitting public health policies to local communities, national governments engaged them from the onset of the COVID-19 pandemic. In this context, FBOs became public messengers, promoters, and deliverers of healthcare services. In South Africa, the South African Council of Churches (SACC) convened a religious forum to align messages across faith traditions and collaborate with public authorities—underscoring the complementarity of secular and religious efforts in the pandemic response (WCC, 2021).

To combat hesitancy, many religious figures publicly received their vaccines, framing it as both a moral duty and a communal act of protection (Sheikhi et al., 2025). For example, Pope Francis and Pope Emeritus Benedict XVI broadcasted their vaccinations to encourage Catholics worldwide to get vaccinated.

National examples were mirrored at the international level by an unprecedented formalization of *institutional partnerships* between public health bodies and religious organizations. In April 2020, UNICEF and Religions for Peace launched a Multi-Religious Faith-in-Action COVID-19 Initiative to raise awareness of the impacts of the pandemic on the world's youngest citizens. Concretely, the initiative resulted in the enhancement of health authorities' guidance, the adaptation of faith ceremonies, the promotion of a greater focus on hygiene, dialogue and engagement, the fight of any form of discrimination, and provision of care and support (UNICEF, 2020).

In December 2020, the Vatican's COVID-19 Commission and the Pontifical Academy for Life issued a declaration titled Vaccines for All, calling for equitable vaccine access and inspiring the World Jewish Congress to issue a parallel statement (Vatican COVID-19 Commission & Pontifical Academy for Life). Finally, the WHO itself developed the WHO Faith Engagement Strategy and launched the WHO Faith Network in 2022, with the purpose of systemically partnering with FBOs in community health education and emergency response settings (WHO, 2021b). *Faith communities are trusted sources of support, comfort, guidance and information; they are advocates for justice and equity and are health service providers in many places across the globe*said WHO Director General, Dr. Tedros Adhanom Ghebreyesus (WHO, 2021a).

3 Faith and Meaning in Health Emergencies

During the Ebola outbreak, the role of religious leaders became most visible when misinformation and resistance to public health measures were most acute. This is because health crises unfold at both the biological and moral levels, where they destabilize *shared narratives* about safety, order, and belonging. Through sermons, religious guides actively debunked misinformation and encouraged cooperation with health authorities. Their influence extended into community mobilization, promoting hygiene practices, and distancing measures. These interventions reframed public health measures in spiritual terms that resonated with local communities, even in a context where fear of contagion overlapped with fear of external control.

A similar dynamic unfolded over a long-time horizon during the HIV/AIDS crisis, which marked a paradigm shift in how faith institutions engaged with public health, especially in Sub-Saharan Africa and Latin America. As HIV became a long-term reality affecting entire communities, faith actors repositioned themselves as healthcare partners.

The COVID-19 pandemic marked the first time in modern history that houses of worship worldwide were forced to close. This suspension of religious life disrupted festivities such as Ramadan, Easter, Passover, and Diwali, as well as rites of passage such as funerals, weddings, and baptisms. For many, the absence of these communal rituals meant losing essential sources of comfort, meaning, and identity at precisely the moment they were most needed (Imber-Black, 2020).

Closures triggered legal debates, as governments were accused of infringing on religious freedom. While some congregations adapted quickly by moving services online, communities in low-resource settings were left behind by the digital divide, deepening inequalities in access to spiritual care (Imber-Black, 2020). Yet even as worship was disrupted, faith communities (i) offered spiritual support through rituals, pastoral care, and shared meaning in a moment of heightened anxiety and uncertainty; (ii) they emerged as vital actors in healthcare delivery. Around the world, temples, churches, and mosques were repurposed into vaccination sites, revealing how the configuration of religious spaces shapes their visibility, funding, and role in society (Wehling et al., 2024).

At scale, these local adaptations accumulated into global patterns. Eventually, evidence compiled by the World Health Organization from over sixty countries showed that faith-based organizations played central roles in health communication, health service delivery, and community mobilization during the pandemic.

Taken together, these experiences suggest that preparedness must account not only for supply chains and surveillance systems but for legitimacy structures embedded within communities. Faith institutions are not peripheral communicators; rather, they are custodians of meaning, trust, and social cohesion.

4 Conclusion

Faith-based organizations have supported health emergency responses across history. The Ebola crisis revealed how mistrust, rooted in colonial and postcolonial practices, still obstructs the implementation of health programs. However, it also demonstrated FBOs' role in bridging the divide between governments, healthcare professionals, and communities. By the time of COVID-19, faith leaders had become partners in international health governance. While this draws a gradual rebalancing of the relationship between religious and health authorities, it also underlines the increasing acknowledgment over the essential role FBOs have in emergency response.

Across cases, one lesson recurs with clarity: timing matters. Inviting faith leaders into public health response only once a crisis peaks limits their ability to build trust and shape behavior. Early involvement in preparedness planning, risk communication, and simulation exercises allows interventions to resonate culturally and ethically. Reflecting this recognition, the World Health Organization recommends mapping religious infrastructure, involving faith leaders in coordination, and providing training in risk communication and health protocols. Preparedness frameworks similarly underscore the need for written plans, reliable communication channels, and coordination with local authorities to counter misinformation and promote preventive behaviors such as vaccination and hygiene.

Looking forward, health systems are increasingly urged to map faith assets, leaders, and places of worship that can be mobilized in crises. Governments are encouraged to establish interfaith response platforms and support training for clergy in epidemiology, communication, and trauma-informed care. Including faith-based organizations in national task forces ensures their perspectives shape decision making rather than reacting after the fact. Across all these efforts, mental health support must remain central. In moments of crisis, faith communities are often among the first places people turn to make sense of loss, fear, and disruption. Recognizing and strengthening this role is essential to sustaining social cohesion and human dignity when systems are under strain.

References

Abdullahi, A. A. (2011). Trends and challenges of traditional medicine in Africa. *African journal of traditional, complementary, and alternative medicines: AJTCAM*, *8*(5 Suppl), 115–123. https://doi.org/10.4314/ajtcam.v8i5S.5

Adams, S. O., Yahaya, H. U., & Mohammed, T. (2023). Cluster analysis of HIV/AIDs incidence in Sub-Saharan Africa (1990–2018). *International Journal of Epidemiology and Health Sciences*, *4*(Continuous), e701311. https://doi.org/10.51757/IJEHS.4.2023.701311

Amster, E. J. (2022). The past, present and future of race and colonialism in medicine. *CMAJ: Canadian Medical Association journal, 194*(20), E708–E710. https://doi.org/10.1503/cmaj.212103

Anoko, J., & Henry, D. (2020). Balancing burial rituals with public health demands during the 2014 Guinean Ebola epidemic. SSHAP Case Study. 8, UNICEF, IDS and Anthrologica.

Armstrong, M. (2021). *The uneven Covid-19 Vaccine rollout*. https://www.statista.com/chart/25832/share-fully-vaccinated-covid-by-world-region/. Accessed 18 February 2026.

Arthur, R. F., Horng, L. M., Tandanpolie, A. F., Gilstad, J. R., Tantum, L. K., & Luby, S. P. (2023). The lasting influence of Ebola: a qualitative study of community-level behaviors, trust, and perceptions three years after the 2014–16 Ebola epidemic in Liberia. *BMC Public Health, 23,* 682. https://doi.org/10.1186/s12889-023-15559-1

Azia, I. N., Nyembezi, A., Carelse, S., & Mukumbang, F. C. (2023). Understanding the role of religious beliefs in adherence to antiretroviral therapy among Pentecostal Christians living with HIV in sub-Saharan Africa: A scoping review. *BMC Public Health, 23*, 1768. https://doi.org/10.1186/s12889-023-16616-5

Bedson, J., Jalloh, M. F., Pedi, D., Bah, S., Owen, K., Oniba, A., Sangarie, M., Fofanah, J. S., Jalloh, M. B., Sengeh, P., & Skrip, L. (2020). Community engagement in outbreak response: Lessons from the 2014–2016 Ebola outbreak in Sierra Leone. *BMJ Global Health, 5*, Article e002145. https://doi.org/10.1136/bmjgh-2019-002145

Bell, B. P., Damon, I. K., Jernigan, D. B et al. (2016). Overview, control strategies, and lessons learned in the cdc response to the 2014–2016 Ebola Epidemic. *Morbidity and Mortality Weekly Report, 65*(3).

Bunson, M. E. (2008). *Uganda: The real ABC's of an epidemic.* Catholic Answers Magazine. https://www.catholic.com/magazine/print-edition/uganda-the-real-abcs-of-an-epidemic. Accessed 28 January 2025.

Dixon, M. G., & Schafer, I. J. (2014). Ebola viral disease outbreak—West Africa. *Morbidity and Mortality Weekly Report, 63*(25), 548–551. https://www.cdc.gov/mmwr/preview/mmwrhtml/mm6325a4.htm

Eusebius Pamphilus. (1703). His ten books of ecclesiastical history. Translated by Parker S. (pp. 119–136).George Sawbridge.

Hoeldtke, L. (2021). *Plagues to Pandemics: What we can learn from early christianity.* https://tartan.gordon.edu/plagues-to-pandemics-what-we-can-learn-from-early-christianity/. Accessed 18 February 2026.

Imber-Black, E. (2020). Rituals in the time of COVID-19: imagination, responsiveness, and the human spirit. *Family Process, 59*(3), 912–921. https://doi.org/10.1111/famp.12581

Krüger, C. (2009). Medical missionaries in Africa. *The Lancet, 373*, 795–796.

Kruger, G., Van der Borght, E. A. J. G., & Rheeder, A. L. (2025). A review of the persistence of HIV stigma within faith communities. *In die Skriflig, 59*(1), a3189.https://doi.org/10.4102/ids.v59i1.3189.

Lowes, S., & Montenero, E. (2021). The legacy of colonial medicine in Central Africa. American Economic Review, 111(4), 1284–1314. https://doi.org/10.1257/aer.20180284

Marshall, K. (2016). *Responding to the Ebola epidemic in West Africa: What role does religion play? Berkley center for religion, peace & world affairs.* GeorgeTown University.

O'Carroll, L., & France-Presse, A. (2014). *Ebola epidemic: Sierra Leone quarantines a million people.* https://www.theguardian.com/world/2014/sep/25/ebola-epidemic-sierra-leone-quarantine-un-united-nations. Accessed 18 February 2026.

Piret, J., & Boivin, G. (2021). Pandemics throughout History. *Frontiers in Microbiology, 11*, Article 631736. https://doi.org/10.3389/fmicb.2020.631736

Sheikhi, R. A., Heidari, M., & Doosti, P. (2025). The role of religious leaders in the acceptance of COVID-19 vaccinations: A systematic review. *BMC Public Health, 25*, 2683. https://doi.org/10.1186/s12889-025-23947-y

The Lancet. (2004). *Tropical medicine: a brittle tool of the new imperialism* (vol. 363). http://www.thelancet.com. Accessed 18 February 2026.

Uganda Aids Commission. (2023). *Mid-term review of the national HIV and AIDS strategic plan 2020/21–2024/25.*

UNAIDS. (2006). *A faith-based response to HIV in southern Africa.* https://www.unaids.org/en/resources/presscentre/featurestories/2006/december/20061220faithbasedresponse. Accessed 18 February 2026.

UNAIDS. (2015). *UNAIDS and PEPFAR launch faith initiative.* https://www.unaids.org/en/resources/presscentre/featurestories/2015/october/20150930_PEPFAR_FBO. Accessed 18 February 2026.

UNAIDS. (2020). *Strengthening the role of faith-based organizations in the HIV response.* https://www.unaids.org/en/resources/presscentre/featurestories/2020/august/20200811_faith-and-hiv. Accessed 18 February 2026.

UNICEF, Religion For Peace. (2020). *Launch of global multi-religious faith-in-action Covid-19 initiative.* https://www.unicef.org/press-releases/launch-global-multi-religious-faith-action-covid-19-initiative. Accessed 18 February 2026.

Vatican Covid-19 Commission & Pontifical Academy for Life. Vaccine for all. 20 points for a fairer and healthier world. https://www.vatican.va/roman_curia/pontifical_academies/acdlife/documents/rc_pont-acd_life_doc_20201229_covid19-vaccinopertuttti_en.html. Accessed 18 February 2026.

Waxman, O. B. (2020). *Celebrating Easter and Passover during pandemics of the past.* https://time.com/5815551/passover-easter-coronavirus-history/. Accessed 18 February 2026.

Wehling, H., Weston, D., Hall, C., et al. (2024). Use of UK faith Centre as a COVID-19 community vaccination clinic: Exploring a potential model for community-based health care delivery. *Postgraduate Medical Journal, 100*(1188), 751–759. https://doi.org/10.1093/postmj/qgae028

World Council of Churches. (2021). *South African religious forum issues statement on COVID-19.* https://www.oikoumene.org/news/south-african-religious-forum-issues-statement-on-covid-19. Accessed 18 February 2026.

World Health Organization. (n.d.). *Ebola outbreak 2014–2016—West Africa.* https://www.who.int/emergencies/situations/ebola-outbreak-2014-2016-West-Africa. Accessed 18 February 2026.

World Health Organization. (2000). *General guidelines for methodologies on research and evaluation of traditional medicine.* https://www.who.int/publications/i/item/9789241506090. Accessed 18 February 2026.

World Health Organization. (2020). *Archived: WHO Timeline—COVID-19.* https://www.who.int/news/item/27-04-2020-who-timeline---covid-19. Accessed 18 February 2026.

World Health Organization. (2021a). *WHO director-general and global faith leaders high-level dialogue on COVID-19.* https://www.who.int/news-room/feature-stories/detail/who-director-general-and-global-faith-leaders-high-level-dialogue-on-covid-19. Accessed 18 February 2026.

World Health Organization. (2021b). *World Health Organization strategy for engaging religious leaders, faith-based organizations and faith communities in health emergencies.* https://www.who.int/activities/strengthening-partnerships-with-the-faith-community. Accessed 18 February 2026.

World Health Organization. (2023). *COVID-19 cases, WHO COVID-19 dashboard.* https://data.who.int/dashboards/covid19/more-resources. Accessed 18 February 2026.

Religion and Mental Health Transitions

1 Introduction

Building on Foucault's Madness and Civilization (1988), Porter (2002) does great work in conceptualizing mental illness as a cultural construct, and a product of the sane's freedom and control. In this perspective, discussing how religious institutions have defined and responded to mental illness throughout history reflects their influence over societies, while the positive and negative outcomes of their engagement on mental health offer insightful inputs for future partnerships in the field.

This chapter traces the evolution of how mental illness and mental health have been understood, from early religious interpretations to contemporary psychosocial models. We examine the role of religion in shaping responses to mental illness, presenting evidence of its detrimental and positive benefits for wellness. Finally, we point to effective partnerships that bridge science and spirituality in the service of human flourishing.

2 The Concept of Mental Illness Over Time

The Babylonians and, later, the Assyrians and the Egyptians held that divine curses were the explanation of major natural events, such as floods and droughts; similarly, certain disturbances of people's mood and behavior were believed to be caused by the action of *supranatural forces* (gods, spirits, demons) on mortals. The Archaic Greeks also understood men as at mercy of external forces (e.g., fate) (Porter, 2002).

Eventually, it was in the elite philosophical and medical thought of Classical Greece that madness started to be conceptualized as coming from within: in making man the measure of all things, they plucked madness from the heavens, and humanized it (Porter, 2002). In that period, the development of Greek medicine led to a natural understanding of mental illness; thus, someone with a sanguine temperament

R. Bedi et al., *Faith Communities and Global Health*,
SpringerBriefs in Public Health, https://doi.org/10.1007/978-3-032-29417-3_5

was believed to have too much blood, and someone with an acid tongue was thought to suffer from an excess of yellow bile. Such imbalances were capable of prevention and correction under that period (Porter, 2002).

While medicine gained intellectual authority over time, it never displaced religion from everyday life. As different explanatory systems coexisted, in the Early Middle Ages Christianity continued to understand mental illness as God-related. The Holy and the Devil battled for human souls; thus, madness could be interpreted ambivalently: as a blessing—when experiences such as prophecy or the stigmata were understood as signs of divine choosing—or as a curse—when madness was taken to signal demonic possession. Derangement was more commonly viewed as a diabolic illness and thought to be spread by witches—women whose speech and behavior were uncontrolled—and heretics—religious adversaries, who could be criminally persecuted (Porter, 2002).

Influenced by these principles, throughout the High Middle Ages writers continued to depict madness as the crisis of the *sinner*. It was when Anglican leaders questioned these supposed instances of demonic possession, fearing they would play in favor of the Papists and Puritans, that the Anglican Church ceased to make use of exorcism. As a counter explanation to derangement, physicians developed the concept of hysteria; the shift was more legal than practical, as hysterical women continued to be stigmatized in practice (Porter, 2002).

A decisive re-centering of the rational individual, built on Classical Greece's discoveries, came in the Early Modern period with Descartes, Hobbes, and Locke. The former theorized humans to be a combination of rational, immaterial mind and mechanical body; thus, madness arose from a body or brain disruption. Subsequent productions rejected the innate rationality of men, to categorize mental disorders as mechanic and sensory defects, which resulted in wrong perceptions of the environment (Porter, 2002).

In the Enlightenment, madness first stopped being understood as a moral failure, and started to be associated with *irrationality*; this link strengthened throughout the nineteenth century, when Gray believed insanity to be a form of neurological disease, and thus a scientific matter, which could sometimes result in immoral and violent acts, often perceived in relation to religion. This interpretation was acknowledged by Churches (Boyer, 2014), which continued to underline the moral implications of certain forms of mental illness, as well as to advocate for compassion and empathy toward the ill (Scull, 2015).

Against this backdrop, religious beliefs, once central explanatory frameworks, were pathologized as delusional and, subsequently, as mental projections satisfying neurotic needs. The limits of this interpretation became apparent over the course of the twentieth century, when mental conditions started to be theorized as individual responses to development and trauma. By the end of the period, mental illness comprised personal psychological processes, as well as biological vulnerability and social environments. Within this context, religion and spirituality were partially re-rehabilitated as resources for coping, resilience, and recovery (Porter, 2002).

How to Cure Mental Illness

Until the High Middle Ages, most of the mentally ill were treated as patients domestically, while a visible malevolent minority was processed as offenders. For the former, treatments consisted of medical regimens—diet, bloodletting, purges, herbal remedies—and/ or religious rituals (e.g., exorcism), while witches and heretics could be criminalized and sometimes faced imprisonment, torture, and execution (Porter, 2002).

It was only toward the end of the Middle Ages that, inspired by the Christian duty of charity, more formal segregations began to emerge; such institutions developed gradually, largely as a result of religious and community initiatives rather than active state planning. Growing surplus of wealth encouraged populations to buy services which once had been provided at home, among which care for the mentally ill. Eventually, the presence of doctors in *asylums*—the facilities designed to provide care and confinement for people with mental disorders, who could not be cared for at home or in the community—started to be regulated around the 1820s (Porter, 2002). Doctors continued to be accompanied by chaplains, who conducted worship services in the mental facilities and advocated for patients' rights.

Insanity became to be understood as consequential (to one or more events); thus, regimens were tailored to individual cases and comprised moral treatment, medical treatments, and environmental management. Restraint was minimized in favor of community life, and started to be normed under certifications issued upon medical assessment. While other regulation invested mental facilities—e.g., on the maximum number of patients, on inspections from authorities—the certification requirement determined an exclusion of the temporarily imbalanced from mental care institutions, and a further isolation of the graduated (Porter, 2002).

By the nineteenth century, the asylum system had reached its peak and its limits simultaneously. While psychiatry consolidated its authority through diagnosis, certification, and institutional management, it also emerged as a panacea to the problems caused by demographic change, urbanization, and industrialization. Facilities became the warehouses for the chronically ill, reinforcing long-term institutionalization rather than recovery.

As confidence in the asylum model began to erode, mental illness was relocated away from the asylum and toward the consulting room. Reintegration in society often relied on medical and psychological treatments, as well as community support (Porter, 2002).

3 What Mental Illness is and Ho Common It is

Mental disorders are clinically significant disturbances in an individual's cognition, emotional regulation, or behavior; these are usually associated with impairment in important areas of functioning (WHO, 2022).

At the global level, the incidence of mental conditions was first captured by the Global Burden of Disease study (IHME, 2024), a project promoted by the World Health Organization (WHO) and the World Bank in 1990. The study was motivated by the need for comprehensive, comparable data across cohorts, the creation of a new metric, and the need to inform policy making. The new metric consisted of the Disability-Adjusted Life Years (DALYs) and combined Years of Life Lost (YLL) and Years Lived with Disability (YLDs). Eventually, its results revealed a striking fact: mental disorders were among the leading causes of disability worldwide (Murray et al., 1994).

Among the different types of mental illness, anxiety and depressive disorders are the most prevalent globally, followed by other conditions including conduct disorder, bipolar disorder, eating disorders, and schizophrenia (Wang et al., 2025). Global Burden of Disease estimates indicate that anxiety and depressive disorders together account for 63.1% of the mental health burden, with approximately 42.5 and 56.3 million DALYs, respectively, in 2021. Between 1990 and 2021, the burden of these leading disorders increased substantially, with age-standardized DALY rates rising by 18.2% for anxiety disorders and 13.4% for depressive disorders (Zhang et al., 2026).

According to Liu and Kuai (2025), while the increase in depression among people under 30 can be attributed to bullying victimization (61.8%), childhood sexual abuse (12.0%), and intimate partner violence (12.6%), the rise in anxiety disorders is linked primarily to bullying victimization, socioeconomic adversity, and the amplifying effects of the COVID-19 pandemic on social isolation and uncertainty, particularly among women and younger cohorts (Bie et al., 2024). The jump in schizophrenia—measured in terms of prevalence, incidence, and disability among the global population—is mainly due to population growth and aging (Charlson et al., 2018), while that of bipolarism appears to be driven by genetic and environmental factors, with high diversity across regions (Fullerton & Tesfaye, 2025).

From Mental Illness to Mental Health

During the nineteenth century, in their scientific observations, alienists focused on pathological deviations from the normal state of things (e.g., mental health), which remained thus undefined and unexplored (Doron, 2015).

At the end of the period, the mental hygiene movement expanded in response to the limits of the asylum system. It focused on the prevention of mental illness through early interventions, which supported individual actions for the preservation of health, and gradually shifted care responsibility from the state to the individual.

In the British literature, early public health approaches—which spread after the world wars, leveraging the diffusion of psychological injuries at the global level—supported the gradual substitution of the term "mental hygiene" with "mental health" (Doron, 2015). The broader idea that mental health was integral to health rather than the absence of mental illness was codified in the WHO Constitution of 1946, which defined health as a state of complete physical, mental, and social well-being and not merely the absence of infirmity.

During the following decades, the rise of social psychiatry—which treated mental health as a product of the interaction between persons and their social environment, recognizing that some groups were disproportionately affected by illness—emphasized how social conditions and structures shape mental health. In parallel, humanistic psychology reframed mental health as the concretization of one's potential, underscoring growth, and self-actualization. Together, they contributed to a multidimensional understanding of the topic, later formalized in biopsychosocial models of mental health (Doron, 2015).

Despite these evolutions, today there is still little agreement on the definition of mental health.

Manwell et al. (2015) define mental health as a state that enables individuals to function cognitively, emotionally, physically, and socially—consistently with recovery-oriented and biopsychosocial approaches. The standard levels of cognitive and emotional functioning, which enclose a sense of internal coherence between thoughts and emotions, intersect with physical health to determine the capacity one has to control oneself, and with social health to define the ability one has to relate to and with others. Eventually, the two combined determine the capability to actively choose one's level of social participation and to navigate social spaces.

4 Religion in Mental Health Today

Despite the evolutions on the understandings of mental illness and the development of effective therapies, many communities around the world still turn first to religious leaders when facing psychological distress (Rudolfsson & Milstein, 2019). This is especially true where access to professional care is limited by low availability of professionals and increased use of traditional medicine—defined by the WHO as the set of knowledge and skills based on the theories and experiences of Indigenous cultures (WHO, 2013).

In these settings, *traditional healers* play a significant role in recognizing symptoms and treating mental health problems via methods of praying such as the pastor laying hands on clients, baptism, drinking and bathing in holy water, and providing ash to patients (Berhe et al., 2024). Berhe et al. (2024) report that Christian and Muslim faith healers believe that praying means that the devil leaves the patient for them to be cured of a mental health problem.

People often seek counsel from the clergy before seeking it from mental health professionals (Wang, Berglund, & Kessler, 2003 in Rudolfsson & Milstein, 2019) due to both a greater familiarity and less stigma associated with pastoral counsel (Rudolfsson & Milstein, 2019). Other barriers to mental health care are represented by high costs and reliance on out-of-pocket payments, with often limited insurance coverage. As a result, engagement with religious support often precedes, complements, or at times substitutes professional mental health care.

In settings where formal mental health systems are under-resourced, different forms of engagement of religious organizations have emerged as pragmatic strategies for extending mental health support.

In some cases, clinical approaches are adapted to religious contexts. Religiously integrated Cognitive Behavioral Therapy (RCBT) integrates standard CBT techniques with Christian practices that are meaningful to the patient; these may include scripturally framed reflections on guilt and forgiveness, exercises to support emotional regulation, and an emphasis on commitment and reconciliation when addressing interpersonal conflict (Pearce et al., 2015).

In other settings, inclusion is operationalized through partnerships between health ministries, non-governmental organizations, and religious actors. An example is the Mental Health Gap Action Programme (mhGAP) by the Uganda Ministry of Health in collaboration with the WHO and World Vision Uganda. In this model, religious leaders were leveraged as community intermediaries to recognize mental, neurological, and substance-use disorders, as well as to facilitate referrals to formal health services. The program expanded community awareness and engagement, contributing to a reported 91% increase in awareness (WHO, 2020).

Collaboration may also take the form of sustained platforms for dialogue between science and spirituality. The Mind & Life Institute, founded by the 14th Dalai Lama, convenes scientists, clinicians, and contemplatives to translate empirical research into evidence-informed spiritual practices. An example of the Institute's projects is the Mindfulness Intervention to Study the Neurobiology of Depression (MIND), where participants were guided through exercises that involved sustained attention to breadth and emotions, which were delivered in a controlled research setting over a defined intervention period. The purpose of the experiment was to examine whether systematic engagement in contemplative attention practices is associated with measurable changes in neural systems implicated in depression (Mind & Life Institute, 2020).

Together, these approaches suggest that collaboration with religious organizations can enhance the reach and cultural legitimacy of mental health care while remaining compatible with evidence-based practice.

The role of religious communities in Kenya. In rural western Kenya, religious congregations are centers of community life and psychosocial care (Pew Research Center, 2010, in Rasmussen et al., 2024); their role is enhanced by the limited access to mental health professionals due to geographical, economic, and cultural barriers (Aguwa et al., 2023 in Rasmussen et al., 2024).

In their experiment, Rasmussen et al. (2024) trained some lay facilitators—who were picked from the local Community Advisory Committee—to deliver nine, weekly structured family sessions on economic empowerment (e.g., families learn to talk openly about money), emotional coping (e.g., families learn to express emotions safely), and sexual education (e.g., families learn to discuss sexuality openly).

In parallel, the intervention team held nine, weekly church-leader discussion groups, to help leaders reflect on their roles and strengthen their knowledge and confidence to talk about sensitive topics within their communities.

Outcome assessments, measured one month after each church completed the nine-session program, showed that whole family communication improved (+0.53 standard deviation at one month). The proportion of youth who discussed condom use with church leaders increased by 15%, while among religious guides knowledge and comfort to speak about sexuality increased (Puffer et al., 2016).

This demonstrates that faith-based settings can reduce stigma and strengthen psychosocial support, by normalizing open discussion on sensitive topics.

Positive and Negative Effects of Religion on Mental Health

The effects of religion on mental health are channeled via individual engagement with religion—in terms of interpretation of reality and behaviors adopted—as well as via the interactions with religious communities. The combined outcome, as reported by the 100-faith diverse, medical students interviewed by Sandu et al. (2025), can be positive or negative; indeed, on the one hand, 65% said hardship brought them closer to faith, and 85% found religious refuge helpful; on the other, 41% believed that being too religious could negatively affect mental health, and 56% reported feeling of guilt related to religious practices.

Eventually, Główczyński et al. (2025) explain that the impacts of religiosity on mental health depends more on how spirituality is interpreted and engaged with than the content of religion per se. Thus, adaptive interpretations are associated with better mental health outcomes, while negative religious coping is linked to greater psychological distress.

On the one hand, religion can provide straightforward decision-making rules that can reduce cognitive load when facing complex decisions, thus lowering stress and uncertainty. Confirming this, VanderWeele et al. (2017) suggest prayer is positively correlated with existential well-being and negatively linked to anxiety. Haverkamp et al. (2025) suggest this may stem from the fact that God may act for humans' neurons as a substitute attachment figure, thus compensating for lack of parental care, informing expectations about the ability to rely on others in difficult times, and influencing self-worth. On the other hand, rigid interpretations of doctrine can limit a person's choice of actions, increasing anxiety (due to the pressure of complying with religious norms), and sense of guilt.

Faith practice positively influences believers' physical health. Indeed, many religions focus on nurturing and protecting one's own body through healthy eating habits—for example, Judaism and Islam support breastfeeding, while Islam, Hinduism, and Buddhism discourage alcohol consumption—and healthy lifestyles. Moreover, religious service attendance at least once per week is associated with a 25%–35% reduction in all-cause mortality, as well as reduced smoking rates, alcohol abuse, and drug use (VanderWeele et al., 2017).

Beyond individual belief and practice, service attendance can create predictable social contacts. Faith communities can normalize help-seeking and offer emotional support and practical assistance; the framing of distress as a shared, emotional experience can reduce stigma. However, religious communities may also unintentionally discourage professional help-seeking by privileging individual prayer and associating dialogue with public accountability. This may be the case in certain in Buddhist traditions, which underline the importance of enduring sufferings to purify one's karma.

Finally, community-level engagement promotes prosocial behaviors such as volunteering, charitable activities, and civic engagement, which indirectly support mental health by reinforcing a sense of purpose (VanderWeele et al., 2017).

The case of mass suicides in religious groups. Religious groups have historically exhibited both inward-directed and outward-directed violence. Among the inward-oriented manifestations of religious violence are apocalyptic suicides, where individuals collectively self-destruct. Such actions are grounded in belief systems that rely on a dualistic view of the world and turn reality into absolute good and absolute evil. Drawing on Abrahamic traditions, these systems frame history as moving toward a final cosmic confrontation, followed by transformation, allowing death to be reinterpreted as transcendence.

Within this framework, Durkheim (1951) distinguishes between suicides driven by extreme identification with the collective (altruistic suicide), and those arising from despair within oppressive systems that offer no alternative futures (fatalistic suicide). Instead of treating altruism and fatalism as states affecting different individuals, Dein and Littlewood (2005) show that in apocalyptic groups, these dynamics can converge, making suicide the only viable means of preserving moral integrity.

In both accounts, apocalyptic suicide involves a shift of agency from the individual self to the collective social self. Personal identity is absorbed in the group, and the preservation of collective coherence takes precedence over individual survival.

5 Conclusion

This chapter has traced how understandings of mental illness and mental health have shifted over time, moving from supernatural and moral explanations toward increasingly complex psychological models. Across these transformations, religion has shaped interpretations and treatments of distress in a dual manner; on the one hand, contributing to stigmatization, on the other, promoting compassion and solidarity. These ambivalent legacies continue to resonate today.

Contemporary evidence suggests that religion's impact on mental health is contingent on modes of interpretation, practice, and social context. Adaptive forms of religiosity and spirituality can foster resilience, social connection, and healthier lifestyles, while rigid interpretations may exacerbate distress and discourage professional care.

Against this backdrop, emerging models of collaboration between mental health systems and religious organizations point toward pragmatic and ethically grounded pathways forward. When grounded in differentiation, partnerships that integrate religious actors into awareness-raising, referral networks, and culturally adapted interventions can expand the reach and legitimacy of mental health care, without compromising scientific standards. Initiatives that foster dialogue between science and spirituality demonstrate that these domains can be mutually informative.

References

Berhe, K. T., Gesesew, H. A., & Ward, P. R. (2024). Traditional healing practices, factors influencing to access the practices and its complementary effect on mental health in sub-Saharan Africa: A systematic review. *British Medical Journal Open, 14*(9), e083004-e83014. https://doi.org/10.1136/bmjopen-2023-083004

Bie, F., Yan, X., Xing, J., Wang, L., Xu, Y., Wang, G., Wang, Q., Guo, J., Qiao, J., & Rao, Z., 2024. (2024) Rising global burden of anxiety disorders among adolescents and young adults: trends, risk factors, and the impact of socioeconomic disparities and COVID-19 from 1990 to 2021. *Frontiers in Psychiatry, 15*. https://doi.org/10.3389/fpsyt.2024.1489427

Boyer, J. (2014). Moral insanity and psychology in nineteenth-century America. *Religion and American Culture: A Journal of Interpretation, 24*(1), 70–99. https://doi.org/10.1525/rac.2014.24.1.70

Charlson, F. J., Ferrari, A. J., Santomauro, D. F., et al. (2018). Global epidemiology and burden of schizophrenia: Findings from the global burden of disease study 2016. *Schizophrenia Bulletin, 44*(6), 1195–1203. https://doi.org/10.1093/schbul/sby058

Claude-Olivier Doron, C. O. (2015, January). "L'émergence du concept de 'santé mentale' dans les années 1940–1960: genèse d'une psycho-politique," *Pratiques en santé mentale, 1*, 3–16. https://shs.cairn.info/journal-pratique-en-sante-mentale-2015-1-page-3?lang=en. Accessed September 6, 2025

Dein, S., & Littlewood, R. (2005). Apocalyptic suicide: From a pathological to an eschatological interpretation. *International Journal of Social Psychiatry, 51*(3), 198–210. https://doi.org/10.1177/0020764005056762

Durkheim, E. (1951). *Suicide: A study in sociology* (2nd ed.). Routledge.

Foucault, M. (1988). Madness and civilization: A History of insanity in the age of reason. Translated by Richard Howard. Vintage Books. https://archive.org/details/madnesscivilizat00fouc

Fullerton, J. M., & Tesfaye, M. (2025). Global diversity in bipolar disorder: The role of cultural and social differences with a view to genomics. *Biological Psychiatry, 98*(4). https://doi.org/10.1016/j.biopsych.2025.02.008

Główczyński, P., Dębski, P., & Badura-Brzoza, K. (2025). The relationship between spiritual practices, mental health, and psychosocial functioning: Narrative review. *Race and Social Problems, 18*(6). https://doi.org/10.1007/s12552-025-09474-w

Haverkamp, E., Olsman, E., Ćurčić-Blake, B., Vila Ramirez, V., Aleman, A., Ket, J. C., & Schaap-Jonker, H. (2025). The convergent neuroscience of Christian prayer and attachment relationships in the context of mental health: A systematic review. *Frontiers in Psychology, 16*. https://doi.org/10.3389/fpsyg.2025.1569514

Institute for Health Metrics and Evaluation. (2024). *Global Burden of disease 2021 findings from the GBD 2021 study*. https://www.healthdata.org/sites/default/files/2024-05/GBD_2021_Booklet_FINAL_2024.05.16.pdf

Liu, Z., & Kuai, M. (2025). The global burden of depression in adolescents and young adults, 1990–2021: Systematic analysis of the global burden of disease study. *BMC Psychiatry, 25*(767). https://doi.org/10.1186/s12888-025-07201-8

Manwell, L. A., Barbic, S. P., Roberts, K., Durisko, Z., Lee, C., Ware, E., & McKenzie, K. (2015). What is mental health? Evidence towards a new definition from a mixed methods multidisciplinary international survey. *BMJ open, 5*(6). https://doi.org/10.1136/bmjopen-2014-007079

Mind & Life Institute. (2020). *Mindfulness Intervention to Study the Neurobiology of Depression (MIND).* https://www.mindandlife.org/grant/mindfulness-intervention-to-study-the-neurobiology-of-depression-mind/. Accessed 7 Sept 2025

Murray, C. J., Lopez, A. D., & Jamison, D. T. (1994). The global burden of disease in 1990: Summary results, sensitivity analysis and future directions. *Bulletin of the World Health Organization, 72*(3), 495–509. https://pubmed.ncbi.nlm.nih.gov/8062404/

Pearce, M. J., Koenig, H. G., Robins, C. J., Nelson, B., Shaw, S. F., Cohen, H. J., & King, M. B. (2015). Religiously integrated cognitive behavioral therapy: A new method of treatment for major depression in patients with chronic medical illness. *Psychotherapy (Chicago, Ill), 52*(1), 56–66. https://www.ncbi.nlm.nih.gov/pmc/articles/PMC4457450/

Porter, R. (2002). *Madness: A brief history*. Oxford University Press.

Puffer, E. S., Green, E. P., Sikkema, K. J., et al. (2016). A church-based intervention for families to promote mental health and prevent HIV among adolescents in rural Kenya: Results of a randomized trial. *Journal of Consulting and Clinical Psychology, 84*(6), 511–525. https://doi.org/10.1037/ccp0000076

Rasmussen, J. M., Johnson, S. L., Ochieng, Y., Jaguga, F., Green, E., & Puffer, E. (2024). Congregation leader and member discussions in a church-based family strengthening, mental health promotion, and HIV prevention trial: Intervention. *Global Mental Health, 11*, https://doi.org/10.1017/gmh.2024.44

Rudolfsson, L., & Milstein, G. (2019). Clergy and mental health clinician collaboration in Sweden: Pilot survey of COPE. *Mental Health, Religion & Culture*, 1–14. https://doi.org/10.1080/13674676.2019.1666095

Sandu, C., Mahmoud, N., Butiu, O., et al. (2025). The impact of religious beliefs on mental health: A self-assessment study among medical students. *Religions, 16*(12), 1501. https://doi.org/10.3390/rel16121501

Scull, A. (2015). *Madness in civilization: A cultural history of insanity*. Princeton University Press

VanderWeele, T. J. (2017). Religious communities and human flourishing. *Current Directions in Psychological Science, 26*(5), 476–481. https://doi.org/10.1177/0963721417721526

Wang, Z., Dou, Y., Yang, X., Guo, X., Ma, X., Zhou, B., & Zhang, W. (2025). Global, regional, and national burden of mental disorders among adolescents and young adults, 1990–2021: A systematic analysis for the global burden of disease study 2021. *Translational Psychiatry, 15,* 397. https://doi.org/10.1038/s41398-025-03623-w

World Health Organization. (2022). *Mental disorders*. https://www.who.int/news-room/fact-sheets/detail/mental-disorders. Accessed 19 February 2026

World Health Organization. (2020). *mhGAP in Uganda—bringing treatment, dignity and real change*. https://www.who.int/news-room/feature-stories/detail/mhgap-in-uganda-bringing-treatment-dignity-and-real-change. Accessed 7 September 2025

World Health Organization. (2013). *Traditional medicine report by the secretariat.* https://apps.who.int/gb/ebwha/pdf_files/EB134/B134_24-en.pdf. Accessed 7 September 2025

Zhang, Z., Chen, X., Wu, S., Chen, X., Wang, X., Liu, C., Zeng, N., Liu, Y., Huo, T., Liu, X., Shi, L., Yan, W., Yuan, X., Meng, Y., Wu, P., Javed, A., Alibudbud, R., Shi, J., Sun, Y., Lu, L., & Bao, Y. (2026). Global, regional and national burden of anxiety and depression disorders from 1990 to 2021, and forecasts up to 2040. *Journal of Affective Disorders, 393*, Article 120299. https://doi.org/10.1016/j.jad.2025.120299

Faith, Gender, and Health Inequities

1 Introduction

Gender is one of the most powerful social determinants of health, as gender norms, roles, and relations influence people's health outcomes throughout their lives (WHO, 2021). Indeed, gender shapes what diseases are studied, who has access to care, who carries risk, and how illness is experienced within health systems, which often reflect wide gender inequities.

Religion extensively interacts with gender by contributing to its construction and by influencing gender relations, thus contributing to the creation and management of gender inequalities. More recent debates have extended religion's role to the theorization and acceptance of gender identity theory, as well as the generation of expectations on gender expression.

This chapter examines the dual role of faith in shaping the interaction of gender and health, sometimes reinforcing inequities, sometimes supporting equity. The tension between positive and negative contributions is central to understanding how religion influences the health of disadvantaged groups within the gender dialogue, and how religious communities can be part of the problem, as much as the solution.

2 Defining Sex and Gender

The phenomenon of sex is rooted in sexual reproduction, the process by which new individuals are produced from two parents belonging to two different classes, called "females" and "males," which perform different reproductive roles. Each human contributes a halved amount of their genetic material, which is brought together to generate a new and genetically unique individual (Sullivan & Todd, 2024).

R. Bedi et al., *Faith Communities and Global Health*, SpringerBriefs in Public Health,
https://doi.org/10.1007/978-3-032-29417-3_6

Thus, sex can be defined as a biological category grounded in reproductive function, immutable and binary. While atypical development of reproductive anatomy—and, consequently, function—can occur, such condition constitutes disorders of sex development (DSDs). Having only two sexes allows the identification and recognition of two different classes of sexed experiences and needs; for example, only men can get prostate cancer, and only women can breastfeed (Sullivan & Todd, 2024).

Sex inequalities do not inevitably turn into inequities, which thus are external to sex and pertain to gender. We define *gender* as a socially and politically constructed set of roles, norms, and expectations imposed on individuals on the basis of their biological sex. For example, girls may be expected to play with "feminine" toys like dolls, while boys may be encouraged to play with "masculine" toys like guns, although both sexes are capable of playing with both or neither (Sullivan & Todd, 2024).

Gender restricts both females and males to a widely recognized set of attitudes and behaviors in a hierarchical manner. Feminine tasks and roles are generally granted less value (in terms of money and/or status) than masculine ones; this stems from the interaction between the activities themselves and the sex that is expected to perform them. Indeed, even if women undertake roles that are considered to be masculine, they are likely to be paid and valued less than men in the same roles; this shows how sex and gender interact (Sullivan &Todd, 2024). In this sense, while gender restricts both females and males, it does so in an openly oppressive manner only to the latter, who are perceived to be inferior to the former. Discrimination to trans people—those who believe both that they possess a gender identity and that this identity conflicts with their biological sex—affects both male and female sexes, as well all genders.

3 Faith and Gendered Roles in Society

In almost every society, we find that gender ideologies are grounded in religious beliefs and myths, in which the construction of males and females is portrayed as one of the very first acts in the production of human society and the natural world (Sered, 2001).

Invoking transcendence supports the perpetuation of *gender hierarchy* and explains in why male-dominated societies access to literacy, sacred texts, and clerical authority has been reserved to males, who have interpreted religious scriptures idealizing men's superiority and women's subordination: women are less rational than males (Islam), women are more tied to this world because of their role as mothers (Buddhism), women are the cause of men's original sin (Christianity), women are polluted because of menstruation and childbirth (Hinduism and some Japanese religions), and women are by definition private rather than public beings (Judaism). In this sense, genders are not inherent to spirituality itself, but rather reflect historically entrenched power structures (Sered, 2001).

Within patriarchal societies, the definition of women's roles, dress codes, behavior, and sexual norms subjects them to males' control. In some societies, women must have the permission of husbands or male guardians before receiving reproductive care, delaying or denying access to essential services.

The exploitation of religious symbols to perpetuate hierarchy is evident in many Middle Eastern societies, where family honor—symbolized by female virginity—can be ruined through the agency of the woman on whose body that symbol is imprinted.

The Role of Religion in Constraining and Expanding Access to Maternal Care

Despite global progress in reducing pregnancy- and childbirth-related deaths, maternal mortality remains unacceptably high. In 2023, an estimated 260,000 women died from complications related to pregnancy or childbirth, and most of these deaths were preventable with timely, quality care (WHO, 2023a). Around 87% of all deaths were concentrated in Sub-Saharan Africa and Southern Asia, reflecting gaps in access to skilled health professionals and emergency obstetric care (WHO, 2023a).

Against this backdrop, religious organizations can expand or restrict women's reproductive options and access to care. In conservative Muslim communities, for instance, restrictions tied to guardianship laws continue to shape women's access to contraception and reproductive health care, contributing to high rates of unintended pregnancy and maternal mortality. Among traditional Catholic communities, widespread opposition to artificial contraception discourages their adoption, even when benefits are clear (Medina, 2025).

Abortion remains the most common matter of contentious across religions: in many Muslim countries, the procedure is prohibited after ensoulment—believed to occur at 120 days of gestation—with limited exceptions (Shapiro, 2014). Similarly, Catholic doctrine has influenced restrictive laws across Latin America and parts of Africa, where abortion is criminalized except in rare cases (Medina, 2025). These limitations contribute to nudging women toward seeking unsafe abortion practices, which are major cause of maternal morbidity and mortality.

Yet, especially in underserved contexts, faith-based organizations are essential and trusted providers of maternal healthcare services. Research in Nigeria shows that women sometimes rely on traditional and faith-based birth attendants out of both necessity and higher trust, despite higher risks of medical risks (Ojei et al., 2025). In Indonesia, religious organizations support family planning initiatives by situating contraceptives use within shared values of family well-being and maternal protection (UNFPA, 2016). In Ethiopia, faith-based organizations helped establish maternity waiting facilities—where expectant mothers can stay near hospitals to ensure safe delivery—increasing antenatal attendance and reducing maternal mortality, especially in rural areas (Gurara et al., 2022). In the country, the partnerships between local faith leaders and community health workers significantly increased women's use of antenatal care and facility-based delivery (Guthrie et al., 2021).

The dual role of religion, whose relevance is heightened by the prevalent role of FBOs as healthcare providers in fragile contexts, as well as by their trust and influence over local communities, calls for careful and bespoke engagement in public health.

Female Genital Mutilation (FGM). FGM includes all procedures involving partial or total removal of the female external genitalia or other injury to the female genital organs for non-medical reasons (WHO, 2020). The World Health Organization estimates that up to 140 million girls and women across the world have been subjected to FGM, and every year about three million girls are at risk. This number has further grown after the COVID-19 pandemic started; this has supported the diffusion of the practice as it has kept children out of schools.

FGM is concentrated in 29 countries in Africa and the Middle East, Egypt, Ethiopia, Kenya, Nigeria, Somalia, and Sudan account for 75% of all cases worldwide (Tønnessen & al-Nagar, 2016). In Sudan, a survey conducted in 2018 shows that 88% of women have been circumcised in total; this percentage stays at 83.7% and 72.7% in the groups of girls between 15–19 and 10–14 years (Tønnessen & al-Nagar, 2016).

Initial efforts to end FGM across North and Sub-Saharan Africa were originated by the concerns on its health consequences on women, as well as the increase mortality rate of circumcised women's newborns. As these worries appeared to be endorsed by local communities due to their religious beliefs, the problem subsequently started to be presented as a violation of women's human rights.

The fact that this concept originated in Western countries eventually undermined its effectiveness locally. Those accepting to see FGM as a breach of female rights, as well as the ones reporting it, were framed as "following the West," and thus were subjected to intimidation and harassment. Frequently, the stigma and fear of persecution were greater than that of the law, which often was not acknowledged locally.

Eventually, laws criminalizing FGM in different regions of Africa, especially in Sudan, started to be passed. In Sudan, the first legal act came in 1946, when the British colonial rule criminalized the Pharaonic version of FGM, preserving the *sunna* circumcision to avoid upsetting the local clergy (Tønnessen & al-Nagar, 2016). Later, many Sudanese states passed provisions criminalizing FGM, but most of these remained to be enforced or involved little to no penalties for defiers. When Article 13 of the National Child Act, which criminalized FGM in all forms in the country, was drafted in 2010, it came as a milestone for the protection of children's human rights (Luigiai et al., 2021).

However, the interventions from religious conservatives eventually prevented its arrival to the Ministerial Council. This setback was partially balanced by the fact that some Sudanese states, like Gedaref, independently passed their own laws banning FGM. As many Sudanese leaders seemed to be more comfortable with a focus on the Islamic tradition and the roles of males and females in society, a final shift in the way of approaching FGM emerged.

The Saleema campaign was launched in 2008 and is one of the main pillars of the Sudanese government to end FGM in one generation (2008–2018). It is implemented jointly by the Government of Sudan, UNICEF, UNFPA, WHO, and the National Council of Child Welfare (Tønnessen & al-Nagar, 2016). The focus is on the introduction of new positive terminology to describe the natural bodies of girls and women. This is meant to contrast the diffusion of the *ghalfa* term, picturing uncut girls as unclean, impure, and unable to control their sexuality. Indeed, as virginity is a requirement for marriage in the Islamic culture, circumcision is viewed as a way of ensuring the girl's marriageability, to increase her beauty and the pleasure for the husband after marriage.

The word *Saleema* derives from the root س-ل-م, which is also the root of words like *islam* (submission) and *salaam* (peace), and means "whole," "healthy," and "unharmed" in the Arabic culture. The aim is to foster the idea that uncut girls are as God has made them, and thus perfect.

Empowered Interpretations of Sacred Scriptures

Today, a growing number of feminist faith activists re-examine religious teachings and laws, and advocate for women's participation in the interpretation of religious doctrine and society. This is especially relevant considering the proliferation of extremist political ideologies, which further strengthen patriarchal structures and instrumentalize religion against women.

In Muslim contexts, Islamic feminism has become a powerful framework for challenging restrictive gender norms. Scholars such as Amina Wadud have demonstrated that many patriarchal rules stem not from the Qur'an itself but from cultural traditions (Khan et al., 2025), while Fatima Mernissi has exposed the cultural—rather than divine—roots of gender restrictions (Malik, 2014).

The Dalit feminist theology emerges from caste-based marginalization within Indian Christianity, and challenges it by insisting that God's preferential option for the oppressed includes them as women and as Dalits (Kapadia, 2019). In Western contexts, feminist biblical scholars such as Elisabeth Schüssler Fiorenza have similarly challenged androcentric interpretations of Christian scriptures.

Finally, in Latin America, the feminist theologians Ivone Gebara and María Pilar Aquino critique gender oppression, arguing that the gospel demands solidarity toward women facing violence, poor health, and economic exclusion (Nogueira-Godsey, 2013).

In African theology, Mercy Amba Oduyoye and the Circle of Concerned African Women Theologians have foregrounded women's experiences, renewing religious meaning from within (Oduyoye, 2001). In Sierra Leone, Sheik Ibrahim Sesay weaves exclusive breastfeeding messages into Friday prayers, promoting maternal healthcare and gender roles built on communal care and protection (UNFPA, 2023).

Though emerging from different traditions, these movements identify and challenge socially constructed roles by reclaiming faith's role in equity promotion.

4 Faith and Relations among Sexes

Gender shapes relations between males and females by functioning as a *primary frame* of how individuals are expected to behave and how interaction should proceed. In this sense, gender guides expectations about authority, competence, and appropriate behavior, subtly shaping who speaks, who is deferred to, and whose contributions are valued. As gender relations are hierarchical, beliefs about gender difference are transformed into status beliefs, in which men are implicitly associated with greater competence and worth.

In a self-reinforcing cycle, gender influences the interpretation of *sacred scriptures*, and religious teachings contribute to the reinforcement of principles guiding gendered interactions. In the context of the American Families of Faith project, Leavitt et al. (2021) sampled 198 families ($N = 476$ individuals) characterized by high level of religious commitment, racial and ethnic diversity, religious diversity, geographic and regional spread, and socioeconomic diversity. Through semi-structured interviews, families were asked a variety of questions about the influence of religion on family life, which influences the public life of members as well. Although no questions were specifically asked regarding religion's influence on gender interactions, the theme was spontaneously raised by 17% of families, comprising at least five different religions. Eventually, answers shared the understanding of female and male roles as built on sacred scriptures and complementary.

Orthodox Jewish women often believe that their role is to care for children and husbands, and maintain the household as spiritually meaningful. In Abrahamic religions, women are portrayed as nurturers and caregivers, while men assume leadership roles. Often, these interpretations have resulted in the under recognition of women's activity, and in an under representation of females in decision-making processes. For example, in diaspora Sikh communities, women practice seva—selfless service—through initiatives such as food distribution, mental health outreach, and domestic violence support. Although these initiatives lie outside religion, they represent a form of leadership that sustains community resilience and fills critical health gaps (Bertolani, 2020). In many parts of Africa and Asia, the efforts of Catholic Sisters remain widely unrecognized, although the organization has established and managed hospitals, clinics, and community health programs, complementing government health efforts and demonstrating managerial ability. Today, facilities founded by religious women remain central to public health infrastructure in underserved regions (Jhonson, 2014).

Eventually, interpretations asserting the passive role of females, compared to the active role of men, have been used as a justification for continued subjection to marital violence. In the United States, Knickmeyer and Levitt (2010) found that some Christian female survivors explained that they remained with physically abusive partners because of biblical injunctions about submission of the wife to the husband. Westenberg (2017) describes pastors and congregations suggesting prayer, forgiveness, and toleration as solutions against marital violence, which compounds women's isolation and delays help-seeking.

Influenced by broader societal movements, religious institutions have embarked on a *revision process* of how the interpretation of sacred scriptures influences the understanding of female and male roles and their behaviors toward one another. Large efforts have centered on infidelity, child marriage, the prevention and treatment of sexual abuse and physical violence from males to females; these have actively engaged women in using their voice to support change.

Child marriage. Globally, an estimated 12 million girls are married before the age of 18 each year, nearly one every two seconds (UNICEF, 2025). Child marriage is a violation of human rights and a public health emergency, as it results in higher risks of maternal mortality, intimate partner violence, school dropout, and poverty. According to the World Health Organization, complications from pregnancy and childbirth remain the leading cause of death for girls aged 15–19 years worldwide (WHO, 2022).

In Indonesia, Aisyiyah, the women's wing of Muhammadiyah, mobilizes grassroots campaigns to prevent child marriage and expand women's education under the religious principles (Fitriahadi et al., 2023). The story of Memory Banda is equally compelling. At 13, Memory refused to marry early and comply to the same child marriage tradition that had turned her sister into a mother and wife at the age of 11 years. Her defiance carried her from community forums to larger church gatherings and global stages, among which the Geneva Summit for Human Rights and Democracy. Supported by her faith community and grassroots women's groups, her advocacy contributed to Malawi's landmark 2015 law, which raised the minimum marriage age to 18 years (OHCHR, 2020). What began as one girl's refusal to be silenced turned into a shift in national policy.

Female violence. The WHO (2023b) estimates that one in three women experiences physical and/or sexual violence by an intimate partner during their lifetime; eventually, this determines increased risks of injury, homicide, depression, sexually transmitted infections, post-traumatic stress disorder (PTSD), and unintended pregnancy, with larger impacts on a woman's life. Violence by a current or former partner is the most common form of violence experienced by women worldwide, with particularly severe health consequences for women of reproductive age.

In Uganda, the Becoming One program trains pastors to reshape premarital and marital counseling; instead of reinforcing male dominance, leaders encourage mutual respect and partnership. In a randomized controlled trial, Boyer et al. (2022) showed that participating couples experienced significant reductions in reported intimate partner violence, alongside improved communication and shared decision making. Similar momentum has emerged in Nigeria, where the Masculinity, Faith, and Peace intervention engages both Christian and Muslim congregations in dialogues that challenge patriarchal norms and reframe scriptural teachings around equity. In a randomized controlled trial, Shaw et al. (2023) found that women in these communities were 61% less likely to report intimate partner violence, while men demonstrated more gender-equitable attitudes and behaviors.

Beyond local interventions, the Thursdays in Black campaign, initiated by the World Council of Churches, invites people worldwide to wear black as a collective, visible act of resistance to rape and gender violence (WCC, 2020).

Eventually, these findings show that while religion has been read through patriarchal lenses throughout history, today religious communities leverage faith and religious teachings as instruments to support gender equity and justice.

5 The Elastic Role of Faith on Gender Inequities

The discrimination generated from gender norms overlaps with ulterior stressors threatening an individual's mental and physical health.

Several studies suggest that lesbian, gay, and bisexual (LGB) youth may be at heightened risk for psychological difficulties. For example, Page et al. (2013) recall that Mercier and Berger (1989) found that 96% of gay and lesbian adolescents in their sample reported at least one psychosocial problem, including difficulty getting along with their family, being misunderstood by others, and harassment from peers.

While among youth in general, religiosity is associated with better psychosocial adjustment (Cotton et al., 2006 in Page et al., 2013), when sexual orientation and religious beliefs collide, in the absence of family support, these stressors can challenge the construction of a positive sense of LGB identity. Though few studies address this issue directly among LGB youth, Schope and Eliason (2000) found exposure to homophobic messages to be more likely for youth growing up in more religiously conservative families; such attitudes contribute to mental health vulnerabilities and discourage mental health help-seeking (Westwood, 2022). Additionally, Schope (2002) found that LGB adolescents with religious parents were less likely to disclose their sexual orientation to others, suggesting that they were less comfortable with their LGB identity. For these reasons, spiritually oriented LGB youth are essential actors in supporting others in reconciling their faith and sexual orientation, by finding complimentary religious associations.

Displaced people are subjected to high levels of gender-based violence, exploitation and trafficking; up to 70% of women are exposed to the former, with under-reporting the norm due to social and cultural barriers, stigma, and shame (UN Women, 2024). Religion interacts with forced migration in complex ways. On the one side, faith can shape public attitudes toward immigrants, fueling hostility and violence. Pertek et al. (2023) provide an example of this by citing Ahmad (2018) on how Muslim survivors of domestic violence in Canada reported being confronted with derogatory comments such as "doesn't your religion allow the husband to hit his wife?". Yet religion can act as a protective factor in migration processes. Many report relying on their faith to adapt to new circumstances, cope with uncertainty, process trauma, and uphold their rights to husbands and hosting communities. Moreover, religious organizations are often the first respondents in displacement emergencies and humanitarian crises. Thus, the failure to engage with religion around the protection and support of forced migrants is a missed opportunity.

The WHO maintains that about 40% of Africa's population consists of people with disabilities (AUDA-NEPAD 2021 in Maseno & Lukalo, 2025). The relation between poverty and disability is bidirectional and contributes to the stigmatization of the latter. In their research, Maseno and Lukalo (2025) found that misconceptions about people living with disabilities included notions that they are unable to contribute financially and that they constitute a financial burden.

Religion deeply influences disability as a social construct, both positively and negatively. On the one hand, disability is often understood as a curse or punishment from God; on the other hand, readings from the Old Testament strengthen the connection between people living with disabilities and God, suggesting solidarity and compassion (Ohajunwa, Kudakwashe, Chitando, 2025). In rural Nepal, female activism in the religious field supports women with disabilities in continuing to seek antenatal care, despite the perception of their pregnancies as a curse (Devkota et al., 2019).

6 Conclusion

This chapter has discussed how religion interacts with gender norms. The same traditions that have historically been used to justify women's subordination to men have also been mobilized to challenge child marriage, reduce intimate partner violence, support maternal health, and expand women's leadership. This demonstrates that gender inequities in religion derive from patriarchal interpretations of sacred scriptures rather than religion itself.

Across contexts, the evidence reviewed suggests two consistent patterns. First, faith can be a supportive to the empowerment of women and minorities, especially when combined with educated medical and political interventions on equity. Second, faith-based engagement becomes protective of women when these are able to reinterpret doctrine and shape community norms.

The development of long-term collaboration between public authorities and faith-based organizations on gender equity requires theological, institutional, and relational change. Faith leaders must be trained in gender-sensitive theology, resourcing women's religious networks, supporting interfaith coalitions, and strengthening the link between sexed needs and public health care. Institutions must improve their ability to dialogue with religious communities and actively engage them in the design, execution, and evaluation of gender equity and health programs. Finally, relations between the two must move from instrumental to partnership-oriented, improving efficiency and effectiveness of service delivery.

References

Alex-Ojei, C. A., Ntoimo, L. F. C., & Adedini, S. A. (2025). Women's motivations for using traditional and faith-based birth attendants in urban south-West Nigeria. *Reproductive Health, 22*(1), 144. https://doi.org/10.1186/s12978-025-02078-y

Bertolani, B. (2020). Women and Sikhism in Theory and Practice: Normative Discourses, Seva Performances, and Agency in the Case Study of Some Young Sikh Women in Northern Italy. *Religions, 11*(2), 91. https://doi.org/10.3390/rel11020091

Boyer, C, Paluck EL, Annan J et al. (2022). Religious leaders can motivate men to cede power and reduce intimate partner violence: Experimental evidence from Uganda. In: S. Schaner (ed) proceedings of the National Academy of Sciences of The United States of America.

Devkota, H. R., Kett, M., & Groce, N. (2019). Societal attitudes and Behaviours towards Women with disabilities in rural Nepal: Pregnancy, childbirth and motherhood. *BMC Pregnancy and Childbirth, 19*(1), 20. https://doi.org/10.1186/s12884-019-2171-4

Fitriahadi, E., Islamiyatur, R., Khusnul, H., et al. (2023). Aisyiyah's role in preventing child marriage in Indonesia: A qualitative study. *Journal of Health Technology Assessment in Midwifery, 6*(1), 25–35. https://doi.org/10.31101/jhtam.2393

Gurara, M. K., Jacquemyn, Y., Ukke, G. G., et al. (2022). Benefits, barriers and enablers of maternity waiting homes utilization in Ethiopia: An integrative review of National Implementation Experience to date. *BMC Pregnancy and Childbirth, 22*, 675. https://doi.org/10.1186/s12884-022-04954-y

Guthrie, B. L., Tsegaye, A. T., Rankinn, K. C., et al. (2021). Partnering faith leaders with community health workers increases utilization of antenatal care and facility delivery Services in Ethiopia: A cluster randomized trial. *Journal of Global Health, 11*, 04063. https://doi.org/10.7189/jogh.11.04063

Johnson, L., & Wall, B. M. (2014). Women, religion, and maternal health Care in Ghana, 1945–2000. *Family & Community Health, 37*(3), 223–230. https://doi.org/10.1097/FCH.0000000000000032

Kapadia, K. (2019). Mirrored in god': Gramsci, religion and Dalit Women subalterns in South India. *Religions, 10*(12), 666. https://doi.org/10.3390/rel10120666

Khan, W., & Arain, H. B. (2025). Exploring Islamic feminism: Challenges and opportunities for Women's empowerment. *Journal of Religion & Society, 3*(1).

Knickmeyer, N., & Levitt, H. (2010). Horne SG (2010) putting on Sunday best: The silencing of battered Women within Christian faith communities. *Feminism & Psychology, 20*(1), 94–113. https://doi.org/10.1177/0959353509347470

Leavitt, C. E., Allsop, D. B., Price, A. A., et al. (2021). Exploring gender roles in highly religious families. *Review of Religious Research, 63*(4), 511–533. https://doi.org/10.1007/s13644-021-00476-9

Lugiai M, Shalabi Y, Rocalbuto V et al. (2021). *Female Genital Mutilation in Sudan: Is a New Era Starting? Sexuality & Culture 25*, no. 4 (2021): 1540–1545. https://pubmed.ncbi.nlm.nih.gov/33584090/.

Malik, S. (2014). Towards a feminist interpretation of Islam: Faith and gender in the work of Fatima Mernissi. *IOSR Journal of Humanities and Social Science, 19*(2014), 25–28. https://doi.org/10.9790/0837-19342528

Maseno, L., & Lukalo, V. B. (2025). Disentangling disability in Africa: A panoramic view from critical disability studies on religion, disability and poverty in Africa. In C. Ohajunwa, A. K. D. Kudakwashe, & E. Chitando (Eds.), *Religion, disability, and sustainable development in Africa*. Routledge UK.

Medina, M. (2025). *An almighty influence: Catholicism's hand in divergent abortion protection outcomes from the Philippine and Mexican judicial systems*. Dissertation,. Loyola University Chicago.

Nogueira-Godsey, E. (2013). A history of resistance: Ivone Gebara's transformative feminist liberation theology. *Journal for the Study of Religion 26, no., 2*(2013), 89–106. https://www.jstor.org/stable/jstudyreligion.26.2.89

Oduyoye, M. A. (2001). *Introducing African Women's theology*. Pilgrim Press.

Office of the United Nations High Commissioner for Human Rights (OHCHR). (2020). Malawi: One Woman's Fight Against Child Marriage. Retrieved September 5, 2025, from https://www.ohchr.org/en/stories/2020/11/malawi-one-womans-fight-against-child-marriage

Ohajunwa, C., Kudakwashe, A. K. D., & Chitando, E. (Eds.). (2025). *Religion, disability, and sustainable development in Africa*. Abingdon.

Page, M. J. L., Lindahl, K. M., & Malik, N. M. (2013). The role of religion and stress in sexual identity and mental health among LGB youth. *Journal of Research on Adolescence, 23*(4), 665–677. https://doi.org/10.1111/jora.12025

Pertek S, Block K, Goodson et al. (2023). Gender-based violence, religion and forced displacement: Protective and risk factors. Frontiers in Human Dynamics 5: 1058822.https://doi.org/10.3389/fhumd.2023.1058822.

Schope, R. D. (2002). The decision to tell: Factors influencing the disclosure of sexual orientation by gay men. *Journal of Gay & Lesbian Social Services, 14*(1), 1–22. https://doi.org/10.1300/J041v14n01_01

Schope, R. D., & Eliason, M. J. (2000). Thinking versus acting: Assessing the relationship between heterosexual attitudes and behaviors toward homosexuals. *Journal of Gay & Lesbian Social Services, 11*(4), 69–92. https://doi.org/10.1300/J041v11n04_04

Sered, S. S. (2001). Religiously doing gender: The good woman and the bad woman in Israeli ritual discourse. *Method & Theory in the Study of Religion, 13*(2), 153–176. https://www.jstor.org/stable/23549967

Shapiro, G. K. (2014). Abortion law in Muslim-majority countries: An overview of the Islamic discourse with policy implications. *Health Policy and Planning, 29*(4), 483–494. https://doi.org/10.1093/heapol/czt040

Shaw B, Stevanovic-Fenn N, Gibson et al. (2023). Shifting norms in faith communities to reduce intimate partner violence: Results from a cluster randomized controlled trial in Nigeria. *Journal of Interpersonal Violence, 38* (19–20): 10865–10899. doi:https://doi.org/10.1177/08862605231176799.

UNFPA Sudan. (2020). First Country in Africa to Outlaw the Practice of Female Genital Mutilation (FGM). Retrieved September 10, 2025, from https://sudan.unfpa.org/en/news/first-country-africa-outlaw-practice-female-genital-mutilation-fgm?utm_source

Sullivan, A., & Selina, T. (Eds.). (2024). *Sex and gender: A contemporary reader*. Routledge.

Tønnessen, L., & al-Nagar, S. (2016). Criminalizing Female Genital Mutilation in Sudan: A never ending story?. Chr. Michelsen Institute.

UNICEF. (2025). *Child Marriage: Latest Global and Regional Trends*. Retrieved September 5, 2025, from https://data.unicef.org/topic/child-protection/child-marriage/

UNICEF Sierra Leone. (2023). Religious Leaders Empower Families to Create Healthier Futures through Exclusive Breastfeeding. Retrieved September 25, 2025, from https://www.unicef.org/sierraleone/stories/religious-leaders-empower-families-create-healthier-futures-through-exclusive-breastfeeding

United Nations Population Fund (UNFPA) Indonesia. (2016). Engaging Religious Leaders in the Family Planning Conversation. Retrieved September 25, 2025, from https://indonesia.unfpa.org/en/news/engaging-religious-leaders-family-planning-conversation

Westenberg, L. (2017). When she calls for help'—Domestic violence in Christian families. *Social Sciences, 6*(3), 71. https://doi.org/10.3390/socsci6030071

Westwood, S. (2022). Religious-based negative attitudes towards LGBTQ people among healthcare, social care and social work students and professionals: A review of the international literature. *Health & Social Care in the Community, 30*(5), e1449–e1470. https://doi.org/10.1111/hsc.13812

UN Women. (2024). Facts and figures: Ending violence against women. Retrieved September 10, 2025, from https://www.unwomen.org/en/articles/facts-and-figures/facts-and-figures-ending-violence-against-women

World Council of Churches. (2020). *Thursdays in Black: Towards a World Without Rape and Violence*. Retrieved September 9, 2025, from https://www.oikoumene.org/what-we-do/thursdays-in-black

World Health Organization. (2021). Gender and Health. Retrieved September 20, 2025, from https://www.who.int/health-topics/gender

World Health Organization. (2022). Adolescent Pregnancy. Retrieved September 5, 2025, from https://www.who.int/news-room/fact-sheets/detail/adolescent-pregnancy

World Health Organization. (2023a). Maternal Health. Retrieved September 22, 2025, from https://www.who.int/health-topics/maternal-health#tab=tab_1

World Health Organization. (2023b). Violence against Women. Retrieved September 5, 2025, from https://www.who.int/news-room/fact-sheets/detail/violence-against-women

World Health Organization. (2025). Female Genital Mutilation. Retrieved September 5, 2025, from https://www.who.int/news-room/fact-sheets/detail/female-genital-mutilation

Religion and Sustainable Development Goals

1 Introduction

The 2030 Agenda for Sustainable Development, adopted by all United Nations Member States in 2015, revolves around the 17 Sustainable Development Goals (SDGs), which rest on a framework that links economic growth, social inclusion, environmental protection, and governance. The broad issues covered, as well as their interconnectedness and their acknowledgment by both developed and developing countries, reflect a building consensus on the *shared responsibility* of diverse stakeholders to tackle sustainable development issues. In this sense, the SDGs represent the institutionalization of Public Value, which calls for public and private engagement.

Despite notable progress, the pace of change remains insufficient to meet 2030 commitments (UN, 2025). Of the 169 SDG targets, only 139 can be addressed using global trend data. Among these, only 35% show adequate progress, while 48% show insufficient improvements, and 18% have regressed below 2015 baseline levels (UN, 2025). The biggest lags appear to revolve around Goal 1—No Poverty; Goal 5—Gender Equality; Goal 6—Clean Water and Sanitation; Goal 16—Peace, Justice and Strong Institutions—while the largest achievements are registered on Goal 7—Affordable and Clean Energy; Goal 11—Sustainable Cities and Communities; Goal 12—Responsible Consumption and Production; Goal 13—Climate Action (UN, 2025).

As a result, eradicating extreme poverty by 2030 appears highly unlikely due to slow recovery from COVID-19 impacts, economic instability, climate shocks, and sluggish growth in Sub-Saharan Africa. Globally, over 230 million girls and women have undergone FGM (UN, 2025); this reflects persisting cultural and legal barriers to gender equality, which complement economic barriers to female empowerment. Education is undermined by poor access to safely managed drinking water; this is especially true in geographic areas with high reliance on agriculture, which is the most water-consuming sector, followed by industry and services. Finally, violence and conflict continue to drive human suffering and displacement (UN, 2025).

R. Bedi et al., *Faith Communities and Global Health*,
SpringerBriefs in Public Health, https://doi.org/10.1007/978-3-032-29417-3_7

Religion occupies an ambivalent position within this framework. While the SDGs are framed in secular and technical language, religious traditions continue to shape moral norms, social behaviors, and institutional practices in contexts where development challenges are most acute. Faith-based organizations (FBOs) operate at the *intersection* of service delivery, community mobilization, and normative influence, yet their contributions are often fragmented, under-measured, or mediated through secular institutions.

This chapter examines how religious teachings and faith-based actors intersect with selected SDGs that show limited global progress. It analyzes both their operational role in delivering services and their normative role in shaping development priorities, with the aim of clarifying how religious engagement can complement broader sustainable development efforts. The resulting dynamic reflects a subtle but persistent governance asymmetry. The SDGs are articulated through indicators, targets, and institutional coordination mechanisms, whereas faith traditions mobilize communities through narratives of justice, stewardship, and moral obligation. Where these languages diverge, operational collaboration may occur without corresponding structural integration. As a result, religious actors often contribute substantially to implementation while remaining peripheral to agenda-setting. Moving beyond marginal inclusion therefore requires not only partnership but recalibration of development discourse to recognize the normative and institutional infrastructures through which communities engage with global commitments.

The Role of Religion in Sustainable Development

As most religions build on the concepts of justice, peace and solidarity, and reach of about 85% of the global population (World Population Review, 2022, cited in Wasserman, 2024), religious organizations are best positioned to address the challenges encapsulated in the SDGs.

FBOs have always participated in global development, and have continued to do so throughout history despite the consolidation of *secular governance* approaches, which promoted a separation of development policy and religion, disregarding the growing role of religious organizations in articulating development perspectives and influencing communities on the ground. This neglect constituted a missed opportunity, which became evident during the "lost decade" for development, and ultimately led to the adoption of more holistic development approaches. Still, the systematic engagement of FBOs in development has been undermined by the absence of shared literacy on their unique contributions within specific development contexts (Schliesser, 2024).

The limited inclusion of FBOs in broader development initiatives has been exacerbated by the evolution of policy frameworks on development, notably the Millennium Development Goals (MDGs) and the SDGs. The MDGs comprised few objectives, whose morally resonant formulation welcomed strong faith-based action under the principles of solidarity and compassion (Karam, 2015). Faith-based groups played a particularly important role in HIV/AIDS treatment and containment, as well as the reduction of stigma around the illness (Sidibé, 2016). The pursuit of the goals by diverse actors was informal and operational, as the policy didn't comprise any stakeholder engagement framework. By contrast, the SDGs adopt a more technical language and show a deeper focus on governance systems, which undermine immediate FBO engagement and often require mediation by professionals, policy brokers, or umbrella organizations. Yet, the goals explicitly acknowledge a wide range of stakeholders, among which FBOs, through dedicated frameworks, formally providing more space for engagement than the MDGs.

Today, many FBOs support the pursuit of the SDGs by fighting poverty, increasing access to safely managed water and food, providing quality education, favoring sustainable consumption behaviors, and promoting climate awareness on land and water. For example, organizations like the World Council of Churches affirm that all 17 SDGs align with their mission (WCC, 2021).

The role of FBOs and religious groups in these areas intersects with the subjects of economics, infrastructure management, and public service provision, as well as with the broader policy field. Indeed, the Heavily Indebted Poor Countries (HIPC) Initiative in 1999, which resulted in the cancellation of around USD 70 billion in debts owed by 35 of the world's most impoverished nations, was influenced by the Jubilee Campaign of 2000, which draws inspiration from the periodic debt relief of impoverished individuals mentioned in the Old Testament (Schliesser, 2024). On education, UNICEF points out that religious organizations still contribute to the management 50% of all schools and 64% of schools in Sub-Saharan Africa (Schliesser, 2024). Finally, at COP28, the first-ever Faith Pavilion framed climate change as both a spiritual and social justice issue (Boorse & Jablonski, 2024).

In the following sections, we will discuss how religious teachings and FBOs support some of the SDGs that have registered the lowest improvements, with the purpose of highlighting how their engagement can enhance broader efforts to achieve sustainable development.

2 Goal 1—No Poverty

Extreme poverty, defined as surviving on less than US $3.30 per person per day at 2021 purchasing power parity (UN, 2025), has witnessed remarkable declines over recent decades. However, in 2025, 808 million people still live in extreme poverty; if current trends are maintained, 8.9% of the world's population will live in poverty by 2030, with Sub-Saharan Africa bearing a disproportionate share (UN, 2025).

As poverty is multidimensional, its reduction is constrained by insecure livelihoods, high levels of informal employment, and slow progress in reducing working poverty in vulnerable regions. Gender and rural inequalities compound its effects, with women and rural populations disproportionately lacking income security and social protection (UN, 2025).

Religion and poverty are closely interrelated; on the one hand, many religious traditions promote renunciation as spiritually purifying and as a moral test, on the other, these same interpretations improve the understanding of poverty and encourage proactive actions to fight it, under the ideals of solidarity and compassion. The Hebrew Scriptures underscore the theme of justice for the marginalized and the poor, while in Christianity their support by wealthy individuals, monasteries, and the church can be traced back to the faith's origins (Holman, 2009 in Schweiger, 2019). Finally, in Muslim communities the religious *duty to help* the neediest is institutionalized by the Zakat levy.

Eventually, while the interventions of FBOs on poverty reduction have been largely substituted by the welfare state in developed countries, in the Global South their role is essential to compensate for limited state capacity.

For example, Mwangi, Kavivya and Gathogo (2025) report that the Kenya National Bureau of Statistics indicates that 79% of Turkana County is impoverished. According to the authors, the persistence of high poverty rates despite government mitigation efforts through equalization funds demonstrates the need for combined efforts including governmental and non-governmental partners. They identify numerous Christian organizations as relevant local actors; among these, they cite the Cross-Catholic Outreach, Caritas, Don Bosco, and Jesuit Refugee Services under the Catholic Church; the Anglican Relief and Development Funds (ARDF) under the Anglican Church; and the Adventist Relief Agency (ADRA) under the Adventist Church.

Eventually, the interventions of these entities on poverty reduction are complementary. For example, the first operates on food distribution, clean water provision, education, and support for microenterprises (Cross-Catholic Outreach, n.d.), while the third targets the youth through education and training, which are believed to support long-term poverty reduction by improving life skills and opportunities (Salesians of Don Bosco, n.d.). This demonstrates that faith-based actors frequently operate at the frontline of poverty alleviation, yet their structural role in shaping anti-poverty strategy remains less visible within formal SDG governance frameworks.

3 Goal 3—Good Health and Well-Being

Within the SDGs, the conceptualization of health builds on the WHO Constitution and is operationalized around four main axes: mortality outcomes, burden of diseases, access to reproductive healthcare services and universal health coverage, and system and risk conditions (UN, 2025).

Global maternal deaths have fallen slightly, although rates in Sub-Saharan Africa and Southern Asia, which together account for 87% of these, have experienced limited progress. Similar geographic inequalities are registered with reference to under 5 mortality rates, which are disproportionately higher in the same regions (UN, 2025).

Infectious diseases remain major threats, with rises of HIV infection rates in Latin America, the Caribbean, Oceania, Northern Africa, and Western Asia relative to 2010 levels; in this area, a permanent halt of funding could result in six million new HIV infections and four million AIDS-related deaths by 2029. Malaria cases have also increased, while new infections of tuberculosis have stabilized after COVID-19. Deep inequities persist in access to essential health services, with low-income and conflict-affected countries facing the greatest workforce shortages and system constraints. Minority groups and marginalized populations continue to experience disproportionate health risks due to gaps in sexual and reproductive health services, nutrition, and preventive care (UN, 2025).

FBOs such as the Uganda Protestant Medical Bureau and the Uganda Muslim Medical Bureau consist of faith-affiliated hospital and clinic networks delivering maternal, newborn, and child health services in underserved and post-conflict regions. They provide skilled obstetric, antenatal, and postnatal services, while coordinating with national health authorities to extend coverage where public services are limited (CCIH, 2021). In Tanzania, the Haydom Lutheran Hospital implemented the Helping Babies Breathe initiative; the program involved training birth attendants in low-cost neonatal resuscitation techniques with the purpose of reducing neonatal mortality and preventing deaths from birth asphyxia, without requiring advanced technology (Vossius et al., 2014).

Faith-based networks have also participated in behavior change campaigns targeting malaria, HIV, and COVID-19. In Malawi, the Malawi Interfaith AIDS Association, in partnership with the Malawi Ministry of Health, the National Malaria Control Program, and UNICEF under the Zero Malaria Starts With Me campaign, trained Christian and Muslim faith leaders to integrate malaria social and behavioral change messages into sermons, community meetings, and household visits. The leaders used a structured toolkit to promote insecticide-treated net use every night, correct net maintenance, support in the recognition of malaria symptoms, and prompt care-seeking at health facilities—effectively transforming trusted religious platforms into channels for malaria prevention, education, and community mobilization (Nicol et al., 2022).

Overall, faith-based organizations serve as critical actors in health service delivery, particularly in regions where public infrastructure is limited. In many African countries, they are responsible for between 30 and 70 percent of healthcare provision, especially in rural and underserved areas (Nicol et al., 2022).

However, religious efforts are often under-recognized, as FBO health workers are frequently excluded from national statistics, which limits their *visibility* in policy planning and resource allocation. This reflects persistent skepticism among secular actors about partnering with religious institutions, especially around sensitive health topics, where religious interpretations might result in an over-moralization of the development agenda.

4 Goal 5 and Goal 10—Gender Equality and Reduced Inequalities

Gender-based disparities directly contribute to broader structural inequalities, which in turn intensify gender disadvantage in a bidirectional relationship. Despite progress on the former, no country performs sufficiently well on legal equality among genders, reduction of violence against women, female economic empowerment, and family life at the same time (UN, 2025). Discriminatory laws, limited access to paid work, and limited decision-making power with reference to women's health decisions are cited in the SDG Report 2025 as the main obstacles to gender parity. Confirming this evidence, the same document states that women are twice as likely to face gender-based discrimination; other exposed populations are persons with disabilities, migrants, people with lower education and economic status. Overall, among countries with multiple survey rounds, average discrimination on any ground increased from 14.8% to 17.1% (UN, 2025).

Religious organizations operate actively across all the cited dimensions to achieve equity among all; as interventions to reduce gender-based violence and are discussed in other sections of this book, we will focus on other aspects of FBO's activism.

Faith-based organizations act as proactive changers of consolidated norms and supporters of the change promoted by their community members. The Side-by-Side Faith Movement for Gender Justice (SbS) mobilizes thousands of faith-based champions across the globe, and has established a track record of effective advocacy work at local, national, and global levels. The group supports the 2/3 Gender Rule in Kenya, which pursues a more gender diverse composition of public bodies, and the Marriage Bill in Uganda, which strengthens gender equality and protects women's rights within marriage (Thomsen, 2022).

To promote equitable, economic empowerment, the Lending Journey—a Christian, nonprofit microfinance charity—offers microfinance loans and entrepreneurial training to women in Latin America. Each country where the organization operates is headed by an in-country Director; internal communities are guided by a community leader, who is responsible for the day-to-day operations and connects with local churches and social workers to provide integrated support to borrowers, increasing their repayment capacity and strengthening their financial confidence (The Lending Journey, 2023). Islamic Relief Worldwide—among the world's largest development charities—supports families headed by women through initiatives such as orphan-sponsorship programs and unconditional cash transfers. Economic empowerment is further pursued through the inclusion of the most fragile in climate adaptation development projects; for example, the installation of solar-irrigation technology in Moyale, Kenya, enabled local female gold miners to abandon their fragile employment, heavily exposed to droughts and floods, to secure a more stable income through farming (Islamic Relief Worldwide, n.d.).

These cases suggest that progress toward gender equality is shaped not only by institutional policy but by interpretive authority. Where religious narratives are rearticulated toward dignity and equity, SDG 5 and SDG 10 objectives gain traction at community level; where restrictive interpretations prevail, development efforts encounter resistance that cannot be resolved through policy instruments alone.

Child marriage in Yemen. In Yemen, the practice of child marriage is rooted in disadvantaged economic conditions, and cultural and societal norms. According to the World Bank (n.d.), since 2015 the country has been experiencing one of the most severe humanitarian and economic crises, which support the adoption of negative coping strategies, such as child marriage. Indeed, poverty drives families to marry off their daughters at a young age, with the purpose of reducing financial strain. This norm is exacerbated by poor female education, which limits female aspirations and opportunities, as well as weak public institutions, which are often unable to effectively translate international commitments in domestic frameworks.

On the international stage, Yemen is a signatory to several human rights conventions and treaties that prohibit child marriage; these includes the Convention on the Rights of the Child (CRC) and the Convention on the Elimination of All Forms of Discrimination against Women (CEDAW). The country has also committed to eliminating child, early, and forced marriage under the 5.3 target of the Sustainable Development Goals. Yet domestic laws set the age of consent at 15; eventually, Islamic traditions often prevail over this formal requirement, effectively allowing underage unions (Nyssen, 2024).

The support of religious communities was pivotal role in supporting Nujood Ali's divorce from her husband. Her impoverished parents had married her off to a man more than three times her age when she was 9 years old. What followed was a cycle of sexual and physical abuse, which led her to ask a court for divorce. UNFPA reports that the judge turned to the local sheikh for support; the latter assumed a central role for the positive outcome of the case. As no provision in Yemeni law provides for prosecution on sexual abuse charges within a marriage, both her former husband and father went free. In a *Los Angeles Times* article, Daragahi (2008) reports that Nujood initially felt ashamed about what had happened to her. "'But I passed through that,' she said, eyes narrowing beneath her black head scarf. 'All I want now is to finish my education,' she adds, her mouth curling into a smile. 'I want to be a lawyer'."

5 Goal 6—Clean Water and Sanitation

Access to drinking water, sanitation, and hygiene (WASH) services has expanded in the last decade, yet billions of people remain underserved due to climate stress and underfinancing. Pressure concentrates across Africa and Western Asia, where high exposure to climate shocks intersects with strong agriculture dependency. Although water-use efficiency has improved more rapidly in agriculture than in industry and services, these gains have been concentrated in North America, Europe, and Oceania (UN, 2025).

Inadequate access to clean water contributes to the spread of waterborne diseases (e.g., dysentery) and exacerbates the risk of infections, also by limiting hygiene practices. This was evident in the COVID-19 pandemic, during which functional sanitation facilities became indispensable preventive measures to contain the transmission of the virus.

Data gaps on water quality management, which concentrate in the world's poorest regions, impede the identification of local needs and infrastructure development planning. While the economic barriers to water infrastructure development in developing countries are many—Souza et al. (2025) cite the high immediate and medium-term costs associated with such investments as a key reason, which is to be inserted in a broader context of macro-and regulatory uncertainty—a key consideration must revolve around the need to pair financially sound interventions with behavioral change programs on water usage (Souza et al., 2025). As noted in an International Monetary Fund (IMF) profile of Benerjee and Duflo, two development economists, *the fact that we think something should work is not enough—it needs to work for the people who use them* (Adriano, 2020).

Faith-based organizations are among the most socially embedded actors in the regions facing the highest water stress and data scarcity, where they *influence norms*, daily practices, and emergency responses. In Kenya, the Anglican Church of Kenya partnered with the Kenya Water and Sanitation Civil Society Network (KEWASNET) to integrate hygiene messages into weekly sermons, contributing to a 25 percent reduction in diarrheal disease, in Siaya and Kakamega counties (Odindo, 2025). In India, the Global Interfaith WASH Alliance mobilized Hindu, Muslim, Sikh, and Christian leaders in support of the Swachh Bharat Mission, helping reframe sanitation and toilet use as moral and communal responsibilities (UNDESA, 2023).

During health emergencies, trust deficits and fear can further undermine compliance with public health guidance. During the Ebola outbreak in Sierra Leone, churches helped promote handwashing and safe burial practices at a time when government messaging faced widespread mistrust (Jalloh et al., 2020). A similar pattern emerged during COVID-19: across West and East Africa, faith leaders partnered with ministries of health and WHO-supported programs to promote mask use, hand hygiene, and physical distancing through sermons and religious radio broadcasts.

Beyond behavior change, faith-based organizations have also directly contributed to water access by delivering infrastructure in trusted communal spaces. In Kenya, Catholic Relief Services installed rainwater harvesting systems at churches and schools in Kitui County, providing clean water to more than 20,000 people and significantly reducing the time women spent collecting water (Odindo, 2025).

Water and sanitation initiatives illustrate that infrastructure alone does not secure sustained behavioral change. Where hygiene practices are framed within existing moral obligations, adoption becomes embedded in daily life rather than externally imposed.

6 Goal 16—Peace Justice and Strong Institutions

Fragile and conflict-affected situations make up nearly two-thirds of low-income countries, where intense conflicts, along with institutional and social fragilities, hinder progress toward middle-income status (World Bank, n.d.). For this reason, Goal 16 focuses on reducing violence (e.g., conflict, homicide, exploitation), building transparent institutions—by reducing corruption, fighting discrimination, and strengthening rule of law—and increasing access to justice.

While the global intentional homicide rate declined since 2015, the number of lives lost to armed conflict has tremendously risen; about four times more children and women were killed in 2023–2024 than in the previous biennium, with respectively 80% and 70% of these concentrated in Gaza. These distressing figures reveal a stark deviation from the trajectory toward global peace and security, and are especially worrying given the effects of conflict on phenomena such as human trafficking (UN, 2025).

Muslim Aid, Islamic Relief Worldwide, and Muslim Global Relief are just a few among the Muslim organizations providing food, water, and medical assistance to the persons in Gaza. Their hands-on efforts are complemented by those of the World Jewish Relief and the American Jewish Joint Distribution Committee, as well as by the financial contributions of the Tzu Chi Foundation and Buddhist Global Relief.

In contexts marked by institutional fragility, religious legitimacy often precedes formal state trust. Recognizing this dynamic reframes SDG 16 not only as a governance objective but also as a question of how moral authority and institutional authority interact in shaping durable peace and justice.

7 Conclusion

The SDGs, while conceived as a secular and universal policy framework, intersect deeply with religious traditions. The persistent gaps in progress toward the 2030 Agenda—particularly on poverty, health, gender equality, reduced inequalities, water access, and peace—are not only technical failures, but also reflect limitations in social reach. In this regard, UNFPA highlights institutional hesitations as key obstacles to the engagement of religious organizations in development efforts and to the recognition of their contributions.

Across the goals discussed, FBOs combine *normative influence* with *operational presence*. Their religious teachings frame development objectives in locally resonant terms, while their service delivery complements public provision. Whether through poverty alleviation, health service delivery, gender advocacy, or peacebuilding, these actors operate as effective enablers of global interventions in local contexts.

Moving beyond marginal inclusion therefore requires more than expanding consultation mechanisms. It calls for recognizing faith communities as part of the social and institutional infrastructure through which development objectives are translated into lived practice. Where technological innovation and policy design are not mediated through trusted moral frameworks, progress toward the SDGs may remain administratively robust yet socially fragile.

References

Adriano, A. (2020). Poverty fighters. In *Finance & development*. International Monetary Fund. imf.org. Retrieved February 24, 2026, from https://www.imf.org/en/publications/fandd/issues/2020/06/mit-poverty-fighters-abhijit-banerjee-and-esther-duflo/

Boorse, D. F., & Jablonski, L. M. (2024). Strengthening partnerships for the sustainable development goals: Engaging faith-based organizations and scientists in youth climate change learning and action. *Sustain. Earth, 7*, 7. https://doi.org/10.1186/s42055-024-00077-8

CCIH. (2021). Contributions of faith-based organizations in health care delivery in Uganda. In *Country spotlight series. Christian connections for international health.* ccih.org. Retrieved February 24, 2026, from https://www.ccih.org/contributions-of-faith-based-organizations-in-health-care-delivery-in-uganda/

Cross Catholic Outreach. (n.d.). *Where we work*. Retrieved February 18, 2026, from https://crosscatholic.org/where-we-work/

Daragahi. (2008). Yemeni bride, 10, says I won't. In Los Angeles Times. *Los Angeles Times*. Retrieved February 24, 2026, from latimes.com. https://www.latimes.com/archives/la-xpm-2008-jun-11-fg-childbride11-story.html/

Islamic Relief Worldwide. (2020). *Adapting to the climate crisis*. Retrieved February 18, 2026, from https://islamic-relief.org/adapting-to-the-climate-crisis/

Jalloh, M. F., Sengeh, P., Bunnell, R. E., et al. (2020). Evidence of behaviour change during an Ebola virus disease outbreak, Sierra Leone. *Bulletin of the World Health Organization, 98*, 330–340B. https://doi.org/10.2471/BLT.19.245803

Karam, A . (2015). Realizing the faith dividend: Religion, gender, peace and security in agenda 2030. In *Realizing the faith dividend: Religion, gender, peace and security in agenda 2030*. UNFPA. unfpa.org. Retrieved February 24, 2026, from https://www.unfpa.org/publications/realizing-faith-dividend/

Mwangi, E. G., Kavivya, C., & Gathogo, J. (2025). Christian faith-based organizations and poverty reduction: A review of Turkana west Sub-County, Kenya. *Jumuga Journal of Education, Oral Studies, and Human Sciences, 8*, 1–13. https://doi.org/10.35544/jjeoshs.v8i2.124

Nicol, J. U., Iwu-Jaja, C. J., Hendricks, L., et al. (2022). The impact of faith-based organizations on maternal and child health care outcomes in Africa: Taking stock of research evidence. *The Pan African Medical Journal, 43*, 168. https://doi.org/10.11604/pamj.2022.43.168.32983

Nyssen, H. (2024). Child marriage in Yemen: Legal challenges. In *Leagle Samiksha*. leaglesamiksha.com. Retrieved February 18, 2026, from https://leaglesamiksha.com/2024/07/09/child-marriage-in-Yemen-legal-challenges/

Odindo, R. (2025). Harnessing faith-based platforms to promote WASH Behaviours in low-resource settings: Insights from Kenya. *International Journal of Arts and Social Science, 8*, 158–163.

Salesians of Don Bosco. (n.d.). *Educational system*. Retrieved February 24, 2026, from https://www.sdb.org/en/Educational_System/

Schliesser, C. (2024). Religion matters: Religion and the sustainable development goals (SDGs). *Religions, 15*, 337. https://doi.org/10.3390/rel15030337

Schweiger, G. (2019). Religion and poverty. *Palgrave Commun, 5*(59). https://doi.org/10.1057/s41599-019-0272-3.

Sidibé, M. (2016). Religion and sustainable development. *The Review of Faith and International Affairs, 14*, 1–4. https://doi.org/10.1080/15570274.2016.1215848

Souza, G., Santos, C., & Lisboa, É. (2025). Water, sanitation, and hygiene in urban areas: A review. *Water, 17*, 2634. https://doi.org/10.3390/w17172634

The Lending Journey. (2023). *About the lending journey*. Retrieved February 25, 2026, from https://www.thelendingjourney.com/about/

Thomsen, J. (2022). Religious actors for gender equality—SDG 5: A reflection on the side by side faith movement for gender justice: Policy & practice note. *R&D, 1*, 119–131. https://doi.org/10.30965/27507955-20220007

United Nations Department of Economic and Social Affairs. (2023). *SDG Good Practices: Swachh Bharat Abhiyan (Clean India Mission)*. Retrieved February 25, 2026, from https://sdgs.un.org/partnerships/action33687

United Nations. (2025). *The sustainable development goals report 2025*. Retrieved February 25, 2026, from https://unstats.un.org/sdgs/report/2025/

Vossius, C., Lotto, E., Lyanga, S., et al. (2014). Cost-effectiveness of the "helping babies breathe" program in a missionary Hospital in Rural Tanzania. *PLoS One, 9*, e102080. https://doi.org/10.1371/journal.pone.0102080

Wasserman, P. (2024). *Global Tapestry of Faith: Religion demographics of the world*. Retrieved February 25, 2026, from https://populationeducation.org/world-population-by-religion-a-global-tapestry-of-faith/

World Bank. (n.d.). *Fragility, conflict &violence*. Retrieved February 25, 2026, from https://www.worldbank.org/en/topic/fragilityconflictviolence/overview

World Bank Group. (n.d.). *Yemen*. Retrieved February 18, 2026, from https://www.worldbank.org/ext/en/country/yemen#tab-economy

World Council of Churches. (2021). *South African religious forum issues statement on COVID-19*. Retrieved February 24, 2026, from https://www.oikoumene.org/news/south-african-religious-forum-issues-statement-on-covid-19

Governing State–Church Partnerships

1 Introduction

In the previous chapters, we have extensively analyzed the role of faith-based organizations (FBOs) in health either as originators of modern health knowledge and systems, as counterparts of a global public health mandate, and as conceptualizers of the meaning of health and the duty to care. We have explored their resilient role as providers—especially during crises—and their influence over mental health and gender debates, contemporary, and yet historical topics. Finally, we have discussed their contributions to the Sustainable Development Goals (SDGs), another less rooted but certainly modern global commitment.

Across these sections, *complementarities* between health necessities and faith-based initiatives have emerged. In Sub-Saharan Africa, religious contributions have been helpful in balancing the strains generated by workforce shortages in the health-care sector. The fact that faith-based providers have a reputation of offering higher quality of care compared to public providers in the area (Olivier et al., 2015) further makes the case for their engagement. In the Eastern Mediterranean region, macro- and meso-instability, as well as financial barriers, is mitigated by the stability of service provision by FBOs and by their focus on the poorest and most fragile—which contributes to the design of financially accessible services. Similar considerations can be extended in regions with variable UHC coverage, often attributable to different contributory schemes. Yet, such complementarities alone have not ensured structural integration. As earlier chapters have shown, engagement with faith-based actors has often been crisis-driven rather than systematically embedded in governance design. The persistence of this pattern reveals a structural gap in how health systems conceptualize partnership.

Moreover, religious groups have been shown to have impressive community embeddedness, stable presence, reach, and trust. Their knowledge of local communities has been essential in both reaching the most excluded and enhancing the effectiveness of public health interventions—e.g., during global health crises. In these same

R. Bedi et al., *Faith Communities and Global Health*,
SpringerBriefs in Public Health, https://doi.org/10.1007/978-3-032-29417-3_8

instances, such organizations have been able to support patients emotionally and spiritually, demonstrating the clear health benefits of religious teachings, practice, and community.

FBOs are in a strategic position to partner with governments in health care, especially in the Global South. The potential of these actors in contributing to public health goals systematically, as well as the limitations of late and ad hoc engagements, suggests that *structured models* of collaboration are worth exploring. Their drafting is a complex task per se, and thus requires extensive attention and capabilities; especially if one agrees that the structure and ability to manage partnerships largely determine their success. We argue that State–Church Partnerships (SCPs) can become sustainable if anchored in comprehensive and clear contracts, incentive alignment, and accountability structures. Because now, more than ever, building bridges between faith and health actors is crucial for public trust in health science and mutual learning (Bazira et al., 2025).

For this reason, this chapter traces the emergence and framing of SCPs within development and global health debates; it then interrogates the ambiguous classification of FBOs and how this influences communication and interactions in procurement and Public-Private Partnerships (PPPs). It then situates bilateral arrangements within the multilayered global health architecture by mapping existing frameworks for collaboration and cataloguing the roles of key global actors that shape global health. The chapter closes with policy recommendations and a targeted research agenda to guide further research on SCPs.

If earlier chapters documented the consequences of delayed recognition—from crisis mismanagement to fragmented development planning—this chapter addresses the institutional response required. The question is no longer whether faith actors contribute, but how collaboration can be deliberately engineered to align legitimacy, accountability, and system resilience.

Brief Overview of the Evolution of State–Church Partnerships

The rise of human development in the 1980s first supported the emergence of *multidimensional* approaches to *development*, which had previously been largely influenced by secular, neo-liberal theories. In this context, religion's role in development became to be analyzed in relation to its influence over people's understandings of what counts as development (Tomalin, 2021). This analytical shift marked the beginning of formal recognition, yet recognition did not immediately translate into structural inclusion. Religion was increasingly studied as a variable within development discourse, but rarely positioned as a co-determining force in institutional design.

As a result, in the first decade of the new millennium numerous initiatives developed at the international and global level to formally dialogue with FBOs. Among these, we cite the World Faiths Development Dialogue (WFDD), the Center for Faith and Opportunity Initiatives at USAID (CFBI), the UN Interagency Task Force (UN IATF) on Religion and Sustainable Development, the UN Interagency Task Force on Engaging Religion for Sustainable Development, the International Partnership on Religion and Sustainable Development (PARD), and the Joint Learning Initiative on Faith and Local Communities (JLI). By around 2010, a scholarly religion-and-development field emerged, and largely focused on the positive and negative ways in which the former contributed to the latter (Tomalin, 2021).

Tomalin (2021) uses the provocative title of *Paradigm Shift or Business as Usual?* to refer to the fact that, since then, FBOs have been engaged in development partnerships as neutral providers able to fill the shoes of any other not-for-profit organization—rather than as faith-influenced, community-embedded organizations. In practice, global institutions have picked which types of religion to engage with based on alignment with liberal values and "passive" expressions of faith. From this standpoint, religions are all the same and there is little need to develop sophisticated knowledge on the diversities among religious groups, let alone to include the marginalized voices along this spectrum. The results are facilitated contracting processes at the expense of the depth of partnerships.

Existing Platforms for Religious Dialogue

The World Faiths Development Dialogue is an independent not-for-profit organization based at Georgetown University's Berkley Center that fosters dialogue between religious communities and international development institutions. It originated in 1998 through an initiative between the World Bank and the Archbishop of Canterbury George Carey to promote understanding of religion's role in development. WFDD convenes dialogues, policy forums, and communities of practice to explore how religious ideas and actors influence global development, contributing qualitative insight rather than direct service delivery (World Faith Development Dialogue, 2026).

USAID's Center for Faith-Based and Community Initiatives coordinates and strengthens partnerships between USAID and faith-based and community organizations to advance development objectives. Established as a formal office within USAID in 2002, the Center provides resources, guidance on engagement processes, and opportunities to convene these groups with government staff around development issues such as health, resilience, and poverty alleviation (USAID, n.d.).

The United Nations Inter-Agency Task Force on Religion and Sustainable Development was established in 2010 as a platform within the UN system to coordinate engagement of member organizations with faith-based and faith-inspired civil society actors. In practice, UNIATF-R brings together representatives from UN entities with a Multi-Faith Advisory Council to integrate religion-sensitive approaches into development planning and programming, supporting coherent policy across the UN on religion and the SDGs (United Nations Interagency Task Force on Religion and Sustainable Development, 2020).

The International Partnership on Religion and Sustainable Development is a global multi-stakeholder alliance created in 2016 to enhance the positive contributions of religious actors toward sustainable development. It convenes governments, multilateral organizations, faith-based and civil society groups, and academic institutions to foster dialogue on issues such as health, gender equality, peace, and environment within the framework of the 2030 SDGs (PaRD, n.d.).

The Joint Learning Initiative on Faith and Local Communities is a global learning network of researchers and practitioners, established in 2012, dedicated to assembling and sharing evidence on the roles of local faith actors in humanitarian and development work. It operates through thematic and regional Learning Hubs that produce, review, and disseminate evidence that informs policy and practice. JLI seeks to strengthen partnerships between faith and secular actors, and aims to improve understanding and engagement of faith actors in development (JLI, n.d.).

The Ambiguity on the Role of FBOS in Health Care

Faith-based organizations are sometimes classified as public bodies, third-sector organizations, private not-for-profit players, and, more rarely, private for-profit ones. This *ambiguity* signals uncertainty about whether faith-based organizations are to be regarded primarily as service contractors, civic intermediaries, or elements of social infrastructure. This determines that engagement follows short-term procurement logics rather than long-term institutional regulation.

We believe this lack of standardization becomes especially dangerous in the context of contractual and institutional engagement, as it undermines the formation of clear expectations on actors' behavior.

In their research, Herzig van Wees and Jennings (2021) uncover that donors' decisions to partner with FBOs are largely driven by their ability to deliver results—supported by their extensive contributions to national health systems—which makes them a good alternative to the government. It is clear that, in treating FBOs as public counterparts, donors not only approach them as public actors, but most importantly attribute to them a neutrality which openly contrasts with any religiously influenced position.

At the micro- and meso-levels, by adopting a *faith blind* approach, donors accept the exclusion and/or under provision of certain services from public health baskets, with potentially dramatic consequences for populations' health. To this point, Tafesse and Chalkley (2021) report that CHAM serves around 37% of the total Malawian population and 75% of the population in rural and remote areas. The provider is largely financed by the government and is subjected to Service Level Agreements (SLAs) which set service output requirements in line with national guidelines. For example, under these contracts CHAM facilities must provide preventive services and treatment of sexually transmitted infections (STIs) for free; yet, CHAM providers are less likely to discuss and encourage condom use, enquire about STI symptoms, comply with national guidelines for STI examination, and discuss the patient's relationship status. Similar cases have been detected in Kenya and Haiti (Barden-O'Fallon, 2017).

Building on Herzig van Wees and Jennings (2021), we believe that donors' and governments' choice of engaging these actors based on limited assumptions should be discussed.

The complex relationship between faith and acceptability of healthcare services has been a constant throughout time—since the very conceptualization of health under religious and moral terms, which can be taken as the very first confirmation that decisions made by health ministers, by physicians, by others working in the health sector, are drawn from their spiritual understandings and beliefs as much as any medical training (Herzig van Wees & Jennings, 2021).

While it is reckless to ignore it, it is over simplistic to take it for given. Indeed, the direction of the influence of religious beliefs over the acceptability of health services has been overturned in numerous cases; for example, the initial stigma over HIV/AIDS has been followed by an active and intense push from religious communities toward its acceptance and cure. In light of this evidence, we suggest that public policymakers should first explore programs providing medical and scientific knowledge and competences to faith leaders, with the purpose of reducing the resistance toward certain healthcare services and, possibly, promoting their acceptance. Finally, we advise for the careful design of contractual agreements with FBOs, which must account for their specificities—and, eventually, leverage them.

Communication Problems between FBOs and the Public Sector

Public-Private Partnerships are often characterized by a contentious communication between parties, whose stances are structurally opposed. To simply put it, while the public's focus is on increasing welfare via public service provision, the private's attention is (often) on extracting the maximum financial value out of the initiative. Yet the clarity around respective positions supports the formulation of realistic expectations on mutual behavior, which can be accounted for in contractual arrangements.

The opposite is true for partnerships between the public and FBOs. Indeed, while their mandates partially overlap, the ambiguity over the latter's role hinders clear communication and contributes to its reduction. Herzig van Wees and Jennings (2021) report that FBOs in Africa perceive to be treated by the government as privates, although they claim they *are doing the job of the government*—which reflects their perception of selves as public entities. Under this assumption, faith-based providers believe they should be actively engaged in public health policy design, implementation, and evaluation; when these expectations are not met, mistrust emerges in the contractual relation, obstructing its development.

These considerations add to the typical complexities of structuring procurement contracts and PPPs. These are defined in most African countries under public procurement laws and PPP sections as written, fixed contracts between a contracting authority and an economic operator, which is remunerated via public payment or user payments, whose relation to performance and risk is variable (CEMAC, 2021). The most immediate example of such difficulties regards the fact that governments often fail to enlarge subsidies, reimbursements, and payments contractually established due to larger budget constraints (Herzig van Wees & Jennings, 2021). To this point, we suggest that further research should explore the effect of direct donors' contributions to FBOs in crowding out the financial contributions of governments toward them, possibly to avoid overfunding some players.

Beyond this basic constraint, there are the difficulties of defining objectives, measuring performance, evaluating outputs, and enlarging payments based on such metrics; a defect met with the lack of ability of FBOs to measure and report operations. A similar dilemma emerges when focusing on standards of quality of care, which are often poorly designed and enforced contractually by the public, and can be disattended by healthcare providers. These challenges illustrate that partnership design must confront asymmetries in administrative capacity and reporting systems. Where expectations regarding data, monitoring, and quality assurance are not calibrated to institutional realities, performance disputes become inevitable.

Yet these complexities should not be read as arguments against structured collaboration, rather as elements that signal that State–Church Partnerships are high-complexity relations entailing significant due diligence, contractual engineering, and risk allocation design. These initial investments are justified by the potential reduction in long-term coordination failures, enforcement costs, and system-level inefficiencies—particularly in contexts of limited fiscal capacity.

Once respective mandates and expectations are clearly defined, contractual arrangements can be constructed around a largely shared normative commitment to public welfare—arguably more pronounced than in conventional public-private arrangements. While such frameworks cannot be improvised, investing resources in their development is warranted, especially in light of the strategic role FBOs already play in many health systems. On this basis, Box 1 presents a set of practical, action-oriented principles to guide the design of durable collaboration between public health actors and faith-based organizations.

Breadcrumbs for durable collaboration

This framework presents the essential elements of durable collaboration between public health actors and faith-based organizations

1. Identify the reason for partnerships: The decision to partner with FBOs must be driven by assessments on the strategic value of engaging such organizations as wholes. These must go beyond efficiency arguments and to include evaluations on innovation, diversification, competitiveness, and risk allocation.
2. Define a joint public objective: Partnerships must begin with a co-defined, clearly articulated, measurable public health goal (e.g., increasing case detection, improving treatment adherence, reducing stigma). Operational, lower-level objectives reduce mission drift and clarify the direction of efforts.
3. Recognize comparative institutional advantage: Effective PPPs assign responsibilities according to actors' competence. Ministries of Health retain authority

over regulation, financing, epidemiological oversight, and clinical standards. Faith-based actors leverage community trust, norm formation, and behavioral influence. Clear definition and differentiation of roles preserve accountability and create the basis for successful performance.
4. Co-design: Early-stage consultations mitigate information asymmetries, enable the identification of realistic goals, support trust and motivation, and prevent downstream resistance.
5. Formalize risk and resource allocation: Durable partnerships require explicit agreements on responsibilities, risk, and benefit distribution. Public actors may retain regulatory tasks, while faith-based organizations assume delivery responsibilities.
6. Establish performance and accountability mechanisms: Structured monitoring systems are essential to prevent partnership decay. Multilayered reporting—covering service outputs, behavioral indicators, and trust metrics—creates transparency and reinforces mutual commitment. Continuous feedback loops enable adaptive learning and safeguard public legitimacy.

SCPs in the Broader Global Health Architecture

The complexity of State–Church Partnerships does not stem solely from considerations on bilateral contracts. Especially in the Global South, such partnerships unfold within a *multilayered* global health architecture, composed of numerous and diverse actors and dynamics. As a result, micro-level considerations are heavily influenced by more meso- and macro-level ones. Global health structures attribute visibility to local faith actors, define public health guidelines, shape financing flows in context with high external reliance, as well as accountability mechanisms. Any attempt to structure SCPs must therefore account for this broader political economy of global health, where authority, funding, and legitimacy are distributed across multiple nodes. Table 1 features a list of global actors, their category, and their contributions in SCPs.

States are core players of international health relations, as along to committing public funds to domestic and foreign health programs, they determine the extent to which their citizens will be influenced by the proposed initiatives of any internal and external actor. The sovereignty debate is particularly salient in the current populist era, where nationalism—in economics and health policy—is on a rising trend.

The WHO sits at the core of the global health landscape. This still holds despite its financial dependency and fragility. In a context of increasing numerousness and diversity of the actors involved in the public health debate, the organization is the only one with the reach, legitimacy, and statute to mobilize the international community and develop partnerships across sectors (Youde, 2018). Leveraging on these attributes, we believe the WHO should issue detailed frameworks for the identification and classification of FBOs, elaborate ethical standards for their engagement, and support countries in the design of beyond-dialogue platforms to practically develop interventions in collaboration with local faith actors. Among the UN funds, UNICEF and UNFPA have pioneered platforms for dialogue with faith organizations on child

Table 1 Global health actors and their roles in state–church partnerships

Actor	Category	Role in Public-Faith Partnership
UNAIDS	UN system joint program	Service delivery; systems strengthening; partnerships
UNESCO	UN specialized agency	Service delivery
WHO	UN specialized agency	Norm-setting; technical guidance; coordination; data standards
UNHCR	UN program	Health & protection in displacement; partnerships
UNICEF	UN fund	Service delivery
Ministries of health	State actor	Policy; stewardship; contracting; DHIS2 ownership
Open philanthropy	Private philanthropy	Grants; technical assistance; advocacy
Rockefeller Foundation	Private philanthropy	Grants; technical assistance; advocacy
Wellcome Trust	Private philanthropy	Grants; technical assistance; advocacy
Children's investment fund foundation (CIFF)	Private philanthropy	Grants; technical assistance; advocacy
Bill & Melinda Gates Foundation	Private philanthropy	Grants; technical assistance; advocacy
Global Fund	PPP	Technical assistance; financing
Gavi, the vaccine alliance	PPP	Vaccine access; grants; partnerships
Supreme councils of imams / Muslim councils	National faith umbrella	Policy dialogue; coordination
National Councils of churches	National faith umbrella	Policy dialogue; coordination
World Bank Group (IBRD/IDA)	MDB / IFI	Financing; technical assistance
Islamic Development Bank (IsDB)	MDB / IFI	Financing; technical assistance
African/Asian/inter-American development banks (AfDB/ADB/IDB)	MDB / IFI	Financing; technical assistance
Médecins Sans Frontières	International NGO (medical)	Service delivery; systems strengthening; partnerships
World vision international	International NGO (faith based)	Service delivery; systems strengthening; partnerships
Save the children	International NGO	Service delivery; systems strengthening; partnerships

(continued)

Table 1 (continued)

Actor	Category	Role in Public-Faith Partnership
Partners in Health	International NGO	Service delivery; systems strengthening; partnerships
Jhpiego	International NGO	Service delivery; systems strengthening; partnerships
Religions for peace	International FBO network	Community engagement; coordinate faith-based providers; policy dialogue
Christian health associations	International FBO network	Community engagement; coordinate faith-based providers; policy dialogue
Anglican Alliance	International FBO network	Community engagement; coordinate faith-based providers; policy dialogue
Lutheran world federation	International FBO network	Community engagement; coordinate faith-based providers; policy dialogue
Islamic relief worldwide	International FBO network	Community engagement; coordinate faith-based providers; policy dialogue
Caritas Internationalis	International FBO network	Community engagement; coordinate faith-based providers; policy dialogue
OECD-DAC	Data platform / standards body	Intergovernmental standard-setter
HISP / DHIS2	Data platform / standards body	Health information systems
Global affairs Canada	Bilateral donor (sovereign ODA agency)	Grants; technical assistance; partnerships
USAID / PEPFAR	Bilateral donor (sovereign ODA agency)	Grants; technical assistance; partnerships
Norad (Norway)	Bilateral donor (sovereign ODA agency)	Grants; technical assistance; partnerships
Sida (Sweden)	Bilateral donor (sovereign ODA agency)	Grants; technical assistance; partnerships
DFAT (Australia)	Bilateral donor (sovereign ODA agency)	Grants; technical assistance; partnerships
JICA (Japan)	Bilateral donor (sovereign ODA agency)	Grants; technical assistance; partnerships
FCDO (United Kingdom)	Bilateral donor (sovereign ODA agency)	Grants; technical assistance; partnerships

(continued)

Table 1 (continued)

Actor	Category	Role in Public-Faith Partnership
GIZ / KfW (Germany)	Bilateral donor (sovereign ODA agency)	Grants; technical assistance; partnerships
IHME / global burden of disease	Academic measurement institute	Data gathering and management (e.g., disease burden)

Source Authors' own elaboration

health and reproductive health. However, dialogue is not architecture. From a Geneva vantage point, the proliferation of consultation platforms without corresponding integration into decision-making hierarchies risks institutionalizing marginality under the language of inclusion.

Multilateral funding agencies complement national financing and capability efforts, with less political influence than bilateral donors. Among these, development banks provide access to finance, support system capacity building, and create enabling environments for scaling up partnerships beyond fragmented projects. Their economic and financial commitments act as a double-edged sword, as they can promote the efficient selection of projects in a long-term view, as well as overvalue macroeconomic indicators in face of humanitarian and rights-based ones. A Geneva-informed governance reform would recognize that ignoring this dimension may produce technically sound investments that remain socially under-anchored. Since the 1970s, the World Bank has focused on health as a core driver to economic development; Youde (2018) cites Harman (2012) to report that the median annual level of health financing provided by the bank between 1997 and 2007 was US$1.4 billion.

Non-state actors' role in public health has enlarged in the last years, largely as a response to rising complexities and limited capabilities of states to tackle them alone. The influence of prominent individuals has been enhanced by rising economic disparities and private wealth, and often goes beyond their own corporations and philanthropies. For example, Jeffrey Sachs' role was a determinant in shifting the tone and rhetoric of the international discussions around global health aid (Youde, 2018). On a similar note, Bill Gates is extensively active on global health via the Bill and Melinda Gates Foundation—which acts as a catalytic investor and agenda setter. Often, philanthropies' lean structures enable them to design programs that are innovative, resource efficient, and output-effective. The Gates Foundation's family planning program emphasizes evidence-based approaches to healthy timing and spacing of pregnancies. As part of this broader engagement, the foundation partnered with Hope Through Healing Hands to promote healthy birth interval planning in low-income countries; the initiative leveraged existing networks to reduce outreach costs and was effective in changing the discourse among leaders in United States and Africa on the topic. Faith leaders were, indeed, trained with scientifically grounded maternal health information (Chenoweth, 2014).

Finally, NGOs and national faith umbrellas are indispensable to guide community practice and enhance the impact of local health interventions. Christian Health Associations, for example, already work as an intermediary between ministries and faith-based providers.

The Geneva ecosystem prides itself on neutrality, universality, and human rights compliance. In this direction, the question is not whether faith belongs in that ecosystem, but whether current governance tools are sophisticated enough to engage religious actors without either instrumentalizing or sidelining them. State–Church Partnerships, if engineered deliberately, offer a pathway to reconcile multilateral norm-setting with locally grounded legitimacy.

2 Conclusion

This chapter has argued that State–Church Partnerships occupy a *strategic* yet *under-theorized* space within contemporary health systems, particularly in the Global South. The reach and social legitimacy of FBOs should not lead policymakers to reduce them as secular service providers, as this strips them off the exact features which make their role so strategic. SCPs are therefore best understood as high-complexity partnerships requiring deliberate institutional engineering. These design features are not bureaucratic embellishments but necessary conditions for avoiding the deterioration of public value, trust, and resources.

Importantly, SCPs do not unfold in isolation. They are embedded within a multi-layered global health architecture in which authority, technical standards, legitimacy, and financial resources are distributed across states, multilateral institutions, philanthropic foundations, international NGOs, and faith networks. Any serious effort to design or evaluate these partnerships must therefore account for this broader political economy. The incentives shaping a local contract between a ministry and a faith provider are often conditioned by donor priorities, multilateral guidelines, data platforms, and transnational advocacy networks. Understanding SCPs demands the adoption of integrated analytical lens that bridges domestic institutional design and global governance dynamics.

Exploring and studying partnerships with FBOs is a strategic imperative. Where FBOs deliver a substantial share of services and influence social norms, the structure of their engagement with the state directly affects health outcomes, equity, and system resilience. In an era marked by fiscal constraints, contested authority, and fragile trust in science and governance, investing in the rigorous study and careful design of SCPs is warranted. Rather than asking whether faith-based actors should be involved in health systems, the more pressing question is how their involvement can be structured to maximize public welfare. Addressing this question requires sustained empirical research, comparative analysis, and institutional experimentation.

References

Barden-O'Fallon, J. (2017). Availability of family planning services and quality of counseling by faith-based organizations: A three country comparative analysis. *Reproductive Health, 14*, 57. https://doi.org/10.1186/s12978-017-0317-2

Bazira D, Aram K, Beasley D et al. (2025). Health and Faith Partnerships to Strengthen Trust: The Georgetown–Lancet Commission on Faith, Trust, and Health. The Lancet 406: 1710–1712. https://doi.org/10.1016/S0140-6736(25)00984-5.

Chenoweth, P. (2014). *Frist, gates Lead conversation at Belmont on 'mother & child project.* Belmont University News & Media. https://news.belmont.edu/frist-gates-lead-conversation-at-belmont-on-mother-child-project/

Commission de la Communauté Économique et Monétaire de l'Afrique Centrale (CEMAC). (2021). Directive n° 01/21-UEAC-205-CM-37 portant cadre juridique des partenariats public-privé en zone.

Herzig van Wees, S., & Jennings, M. (2021). The challenges of donor engagement with faith-based organizations in Cameroon's health sector: A qualitative study. *Health Policy and Planning, 36*(4), 464–472. https://doi.org/10.1093/heapol/czab006

International Partnership on Religion and Sustainable Development (PaRD). (n.d.) PaRD's Mission and Vision.Retrieved September 29, 2025, https://www.partner-religion-development.org

Joint Learning Initiative on Faith and Local Communities (n.d.-a). About the Joint Learning Initiative on Faith Local Communities. Accessed 27 September 2025.

Joint Learning Initiative on Faith and Local Communities (n.d.-b) About the Learning Initiative on Faith & Local Communities. Retrieved September 29, 2025, from https://jliflc.com/aht-ms/

Joint Learning Initiative on Faith and Local Communities (n.d.-c) Learning Hubs. Retrieved September 29, 2025, from https://jliflc.com/aht-ms/

Olivier, J., Tsimpo, C., Gemignani, R., et al. (2015). Understanding the roles of faith-based health-care providers in Africa: Review of the evidence with a focus on magnitude, reach, cost, and satisfaction. *The Lancet, 386*(10005), 1765–1775. https://doi.org/10.1016/S0140-6736(15)60251-3

Tafesse, W., & Chalkley, M. (2021). Faith-based provision of sexual and reproductive healthcare in Malawi. *Social Science & Medicine, 282*, 113997. https://doi.org/10.1016/j.socscimed.2021.113997

Tomalin, E. (2021). Religions and development: A paradigm shift or business as usual? *Religion, 51*(1), 105–124. https://doi.org/10.1080/0048721X.2020.1792055

U.S. Agency for International Development (USAID). (n.d.). *Center for Faith and Opportunity Initiatives*. USAID.

United Nations Interagency Task Force on Religion and Sustainable Development (UNIATF). (2020). Annual Report of the United Nations Interagency Task Force on Religion and Sustainable Development: Engaging with Religion and Faith-Based. Retrieved October 02, 2025, from https://www.rfp.org/

World Faiths Development Dialogue. (2026). *About WFDD.* Berkley Center for Religion, Peace, and World Affairs, Georgetown University. https://berkleycenter.georgetown.edu/wfdd/about

Youde, J. (2018). *Global Health governance in international society.* Oxford University Press.

Appendix: Further Readings

To build on the frameworks introduced in this book, the following reading list offers deeper academic and practical resources. These works help move the conversation from viewing faith-health collaboration as a crisis response to understanding it as a permanent, evidence-based part of global health systems. The field is interdisciplinary; this is mirrored by the list of recommended readings below, which span from sociological research to historical studies of international health policy, and practical leadership models.

This section supports the book's argument that faith communities are not optional partners but essential parts of health systems.

- Idler (2014), *Religion as a Social Determinant of Health*, Chapter 1.

  Idler applies the established social determinants of health framework to religion, helping move faith-based health discussions into mainstream policy conversations. She explains specific mechanisms, such as social support, social control, and social capital, that clarify why faith networks are often resilient and effective.
- Idler et al. (2019), Partnerships Between Public Health Agencies and Faith Communities.

  This editorial addresses the "systematic marginalization" discussed in our chapters. It outlines evidence-based best practices for State–Church Partnerships, including prioritizing community-driven ("ground-up") approaches and managing ideological differences.
- Brown (2014), *Religion and Global Health*, in Idler, ed., 2014.

  Expanding on the scale of faith-based care in Africa, Brown offers an interdisciplinary review of Christian health engagement in low-resource settings. He provides a critical historical look at medical missionaries, helping readers explore the "legacy of mistrust" and "colonial medicine" discussed earlier in the book.

This work provides the institutional history behind the policy changes discussed in the book.

R. Bedi et al., *Faith Communities and Global Health*,
SpringerBriefs in Public Health, https://doi.org/10.1007/978-3-032-29417-3

- Peng-Keller et al. (2022), *The Spirit of Global Health: Sacred Partners.*

  This book examines the WHO's 2022 Faith Engagement Strategy as a turning point, while also tracing the organization's earlier history (1946–2021). It explains how religion was at times forgotten and later rediscovered within global health policy. It also provides important background on the 1984 WHA 37.13 resolution (where the spiritual dimension became part of WHO Member States' strategies for health) that helped shape the "Health for All" vision referenced throughout the book.

  This section expands on the theological and philosophical foundations of health.

- VanderWeele (2024), *A Theology of Health: Wholeness and Human Flourishing.*

  VanderWeele offers a systematic theological framework for understanding health. He distinguishes between "health of the body" (normal functioning) and "health of the person" (flourishing and communion with God). He defines flourishing as a state where all aspects of life, physical, mental, social, and spiritual are good as intended by God. This connects to the expanded "WHO+" definition discussed in the book, emphasizing that spiritual well-being provides meaning and hope that support resilience.

Building on the mapping and collaboration strategies discussed in this book, these readings provide practical tools and methods.

- Cochrane, McFarland, and Gunderson (2014), Chapter 23 (in Idler, ed., 2014).

  This chapter introduces the PIRHANA tool (Participatory Inquiry into Religious Health Assets, Networks, and Agency), which supports systematic mapping of faith-based health initiatives. It distinguishes between tangible assets (hospitals, clinics, staff) and intangible assets (trust, motivation, reach, vocation). The authors also propose Reverse epidemiology which shifts attention from disease and risk factors to the strengths and life-giving resources that promote health in communities. Instead of focusing only on pathology, it highlights trust, relationships, meaning, and social support as sources of resilience. It prioritizes people's lived experiences of health ("healthworlds") alongside biomedical data.
- Idler et al. (2019), Partnerships Between Public Health Agencies and Faith Communities.

  This editorial directly addresses the "systematic marginalization" discussed in our book by shifting the focus from personal religious belief to the collective influence and institutional strength of faith communities. It outlines essential "best practices" for the State–Church Partnerships proposed, such as prioritizing a ground-up approach, respecting domain expertise, and recognizing faith leaders as change agents rather than obstacles.

For those implementing shared leadership models, these works provide guidance for internal organizational change.

- Roxburgh and Romanuk (2006), *The Missional Leader: Equipping Your Church to Reach a Changing World.*

  The authors go further than our book's focus on external partnerships by detailing the internal cultural shift required within religious organizations to engage with a modern, rapidly changing global landscape. It describes a shift from a "Pastoral Model," where leaders primarily maintain and fix problems, to a "Missional Model," where leaders cultivate a shared imagination that engages changing contexts. The authors' Three Zone Model of Missional Leadership helps leaders identify whether their organization is emergent (innovative), performative (stable and maintaining), or reactive (in crisis) especially in times of disruptive change requiring new leadership capacities. They also recommend tools such as 360-degree feedback and accountable leadership teams to support long-term change. This tool which collects feedback from a cross-section of people, including staff, church members, peers, board members, and supervisors is designed to provide a "photograph" of how others perceive a leader's functioning across various missional readiness factors

These readings deepen the book's case studies on Ebola, HIV/AIDS, and COVID-19 by examining religion's complex influence.

- Blevins et al. (2019), Faith and Global Health Practice in Ebola and HIV Emergencies.

  This article highlights how health interventions can fail when they ignore the cultural and spiritual practices communities use to make sense of death. It highlights how religious leaders helped adapt burial rites during Ebola to make them both safe and dignified. The authors describe religion as "double-edged," capable of either increasing stigma or promoting public health compliance.
- Dalmida and Thurman (2014), HIV/AIDS (in Idler, ed., 2014).

  Chapter 24 explores the paradox of religious institutions providing compassionate care discussed in our book while also reinforcing moral tensions around prevention methods such as condom use. It traces how religious communities became key providers of psychosocial support as HIV shifted from an acute to a chronic condition.
- Peng-Keller et al. (2022), *The Spirit of Global Health: WHO and Religious Actors During COVID-19.*

  This work examines the WHO's collaboration with religious leaders during the COVID-19 pandemic, including the EPI-WIN network. It details how the WHO consulted with religious actors to address vaccine hesitancy and medical racism, ultimately recognizing that faith leaders often hold greater community trust than politicians. The pandemic strengthened the case for formal faith-health partnerships in global governance.

Index

R. Bedi et al., *Faith Communities and Global Health*, SpringerBriefs in Public Health, https://doi.org/10.1007/978-3-032-29417-3

MIX
Papier aus verantwortungsvollen Quellen
Paper from responsible sources
FSC® C105338

If you have any concerns about our products,
you can contact us on
ProductSafety@springernature.com

In case Publisher is established outside the EU,
the EU authorized representative is:
Springer Nature Customer Service Center GmbH
Europaplatz 3, 69115 Heidelberg, Germany

Printed by Libri Plureos GmbH
in Hamburg, Germany